The
Sexually Confident
Wife

The
Sexually Confident
Wife

Connecting With Your Husband
Mind • Body • Heart • Spirit

Shannon Ethridge

Broadway Books

New York

BROADWAY

Published in the United States by Broadway Books, an imprint of the Crown
Publishing Group, a division of Random House, Inc., New York.

www.crownpublishing.com

BROADWAY BOOKS and the Broadway Books colophon
are trademarks of Random House, Inc.

Originally published in hardcover in the United States by Broadway Books, New York in 2008.

Library of Congress Cataloging-in-Publication Data
Ethridge, Shannon.
The sexually confident wife : connecting with your husband
mind heart body spirit / Shannon Ethridge.
1. Sex in marriage. 2. Sex instruction for women. 3. Married women—
Sexual behavior. 4. Married women—Psychology. 5. Women—Sexual behavior.
6. Women—Psychology.
I. Title.

ISBN 978-0-7679-2606-5

Printed in the United States of America

Design by Chris Welch
Illustrations by Brett Johnson

9 10

First Paperback Edition

Dedicated to every woman who has shared her personal story
with me over the past two decades.
May this book bring great hope and healing.

Author's Note

In describing my experience with women I have counseled, I have changed their names and other identifying characteristics in order to protect their privacy.

Contents

Part 3

The Fantastic Sexual Female

Part 4

Getting Behind Closed Doors

Part 5

Overcoming Obstacles

Part 6

A Celebration of Sexual Confidence

Part 1

Opening Our Eyes

1

Where Did Our Confidence Go?

At one time, I was perhaps one of the most sexually confident women on the planet. I loved my body. I was willing to share it freely. I enjoyed sex.

What changed? I got married. And it took me longer than a decade (along with months of counseling) to return to the place where I loved my body, shared it freely, and enjoyed sex once again.

Some of you know what I'm talking about. As single women, sex was often a game that we liked to play, and some of us were very skilled at it. *I've got it. You want it. But the price of admission into my private playground is a big dose of attention and affection. Make me feel really good about myself, and I'll make you feel really good in exchange.* But now that we're sleeping next to the same man night after night, month after month, year after year, the challenge has worn off. The payoff is no longer clear. Hubby isn't wooing and pursuing us like he used to, so our motivation wanes. Sex feels more like an obligation than a mutual thrill.

And maybe that mental list of previous sexual partners has begun to haunt you. You calculate all of the sexual favors you paid out in hopes of earning emotional interest, but now you feel sexually bankrupt. *How could I have just given my body away like that? And how could my husband possibly love me and want to be with me after all I've done?* you may wonder.

Or perhaps you weren't skilled at all when you came into marriage. You assumed your husband was going to teach you everything you needed to know about sex, or that you'd figure it out together. Now that he's so masterfully taught you that the round peg goes in the round hole for approximately 2.8 minutes, you're left wondering, *Is this all there is?* Disappointed and disillusioned, you've come to see sex as something you're expected to just dish out like a scoop of ice cream whenever he gets hungry, which makes you want to close the ice cream shop altogether most days.

Or maybe your sexual confidence has been robbed because while you've been dishing it out, he's been salivating over other flavors. You notice him glance up and down another woman's body as she walks by. You know where he keeps his pornography stash. You've gone to his most recent websites to see what he's been looking at on his laptop. You catch him masturbating alone, most likely fantasizing about any woman except you.

Perhaps you, like millions of other ladies, have lost your sexual confidence as a result of past sexual abuse. Rather than associating sex with passion and pleasure, you've associated it with pain and degradation. You know in your head that it's not your husband's fault that you were abused, but you've insulated yourself from further pain with walls of anger, resentment, and fear of intimacy. You can't imagine how you'll ever get over what's been done to you in the past.

Maybe you simply do not feel beautiful, especially when you compare your postpartum body (complete with stretch-marked hips, flabby tummy, and saggy boobs) to the airbrushed magazine models. Excess food becomes your drug of choice to medicate your emotional pain. Your husband asks why you're eating turtle cheesecake if you already feel fat. You inhale a second piece just to spite him, and think, *No sex for you again tonight, pal!*

Or perhaps children clinging to your ankles all day prevent you from mustering enough energy to enjoy sex much anymore. Your idea of a blissfully indulgent evening is ordering takeout, throwing the paper plates away after dinner, and heading straight for bed at eight p.m. without having to tuck anyone in or take care of anyone else's needs.

Oh, the many issues that we let rob us of our sexual confidence! No wonder more and more married people are claiming to be sexually frustrated. No wonder there are so many sexless marriages today. In 2005, *Family Circle* magazine published the results of a national survey in which they asked married women to reveal their innermost desires, needs, regrets, and joys. Consider these results and what they say about the quality of couples' relationships:

- Only 8 percent of married women consider their sex life "very hot."
- 21 percent call their sex life "routine and boring."
- 21 percent of respondents asked, "What sex life?"[1]

Sound familiar? Maybe you've been thinking you were alone in your struggle to discover sexual fulfillment. Think again . . .

- 20 to 30 percent of men and 30 to 50 percent of women say they have little or no sex drive.[2]

- 33 to 50 percent of women experience orgasm infrequently and are dissatisfied with how often they reach orgasm.[3]
- 10 to 15 percent of American women have never experienced orgasm at all.[4]

Although many women have lost (or never found) their sexual groove in marriage, it doesn't mean they are sexually dead. We get married, not buried. If your husband isn't floating your sexual boat, you may be thinking about what it would be like to sail on other oceans. According to the aforementioned *Family Circle* survey . . .

- 44 percent of wives have fantasized about having an affair, most often with a stranger, celebrity, or coworker.
- 29 percent of women admit to flirting with other men.
- 25 percent of women fantasize about another man during the act of sex.[5]

If you ask me, these statistics merely indicate the number of women who are willing to admit their issues to researchers. I think the number of women who actually engage in these extramarital games and struggle with finding genuine sexual fulfillment within their marriage is much higher. What gives me this impression? The multitude of e-mails I receive every day from women lamenting their lack of sexual confidence. For example:

- Lisa, who was sexually abused as a child, confesses, "Sexual fantasies of other men have always been an issue for me, and extramarital affairs littered the first five years of my marriage. Even now that I'm being faithful to my husband, I still struggle with feeling the need to compete with other women for my husband's attention. We spent two weeks in Hawaii and I was miserable the whole time because of all the bikini-clad bodies around. My husband says, 'But I'm with *you*, so what's your problem?' I just wish I knew the answer to that question."

- Sylvia was sexually active before marriage, then married a virgin three years ago. She asks, "How do you and your husband keep the past out of your marriage? Do you ever talk about it? How do you get beyond the hurt? I am afraid this is affecting my sex life because I still feel 'unclean' at times. I am also afraid of trying anything new to please him because I don't want him to think I'm a slut. I know he must think about my past sometimes, but I don't ever want to talk about it. I just want the whole thing to be forgotten, but I can't erase the memories or their negative effects."

- Abby has been married eight years and has one child. She writes, "My husband and I get along very well, but it feels more like we're friends or business partners than lovers. I'm no longer attracted to him physically at all and I can't stand it when he comes near me for even just a quick kiss. I actually feel repulsed by him. I'm not frigid, but there's just no 'chemistry' any longer. How can I find my husband desirable again?"

- Terri came into marriage expecting that everything would come naturally, but it hasn't worked that way. She says, "I just can't relax and get into it. I have too many hang-ups about anything sexual. I love my husband, but I wish sex didn't have to be a part of the marital equation at all. When I give in out of obligation, I usually just close my eyes and think of something else. I know that's probably not all that fun to him, but I don't know what else to do."

When I receive these kinds of questions and comments, I always wonder the same thing: *What difference would sexual confidence make in these women's lives? In their husbands' lives? In the lives of their families?*

Defining Sexual Confidence

Perhaps you are wondering what it would be like to be a sexually confident wife. First let's talk about what it *isn't* like. It's not about having a great body or obsessing over getting one. It's not about fitting the "young, hot" stereotypical mold. It's not about being his sexual rag doll, doormat, or vending machine. It's not about killing your conscience and being willing to do anything and everything to sexually satisfy someone else. It's simply not about becoming someone you aren't.

It's about becoming who you really are, and humans are naturally sexual beings. Perhaps you don't feel like a sexual being now, but I hope that by the time you finish reading this book, you will. In fact, I hope you'll feel not just sexual but sexually confident as you put these principles into practice.

As a sexually confident wife, you will learn to love your body and feel beautiful in your own skin. You'll be content with being the best _____ you can be (fill in the blank with your own first and last names) and not feel the need to compare yourself or your husband to anyone else. You'll come to believe wholeheartedly that your husband finds you incredibly desirable. You'll be able to openly communicate what you find pleasurable, as well as what is beyond your personal boundaries. You will feel great about what you have to offer your husband, and will be able to relax and freely enjoy all that he has to offer you.

A PERSONAL REPORT CARD

Whether you have a long way to go in this process, or just a little, is based on where you currently stand. To help you assess where you are on the sexual confidence scale, here's a list of 69 questions (pun intended!) to ask yourself.

Disagree										**Strongly Agree**
0	1	2	3	4	5	6	7	8	9	10

____ 1. I feel good about who I am as a sexual female.

____ 2. I have no doubt that my husband finds me sexually attractive.

____ 3. I trust my husband completely when making love.

____ 4. I am comfortable having sex as often as my husband wants to.

____ 5. I am comfortable having sex however my husband wants to do it.

____ 6. I initiate sex often with my husband with confidence that I won't be denied.

____ 7. I am comfortable inside my own skin and like who I see in the mirror.

____ 8. I experience sexual desire for my husband.

____ 9. I am comfortable with my husband looking at my naked body.

____ 10. I believe my husband likes my body just the way it is.

____ 11. I like the size of my breasts.

____ 12. I believe my husband likes the size of my breasts.

____ 13. I am comfortable with the shape of my body.

____ 14. I am comfortable with the size of my body.

_____ 15. I am not ashamed to let my husband look at my vagina.

_____ 16. I am not embarrassed to let my husband touch my vagina.

_____ 17. I am comfortable with my husband performing oral sex.

_____ 18. I am at ease with vaginal penetration (intercourse).

_____ 19. I believe I know exactly what turns my husband on.

_____ 20. I have confidence that I can bring my husband to climax every time.

_____ 21. I believe that my own sexual pleasure is important to my husband.

_____ 22. I am worthy of the investment of time and effort it takes for me to orgasm.

_____ 23. It does not bother me for other people to know that I am a sexual woman.

_____ 24. It does not bother me if my children are aware that their parents have sex.

_____ 25. I am very interested in sexual activity with my husband.

_____ 26. My husband considers me an interesting sex partner.

_____ 27. I am willing to try new sexual positions.

_____ 28. I am willing to try new sexual acts.

_____ 29. I feel the freedom to verbalize my personal desires in bed.

_____ 30. I am comfortable asking how I might pleasure my husband sexually.

_____ 31. I do not worry about my husband asking me to do something degrading in bed.

_____ 32. I don't worry about my husband rejecting my sexual advances.

_____ 33. I have confidence that I satisfy my husband completely in the bedroom.

_____ 34. I believe my husband only seeks sexual pleasure within our marriage.

_____ 35. My husband doesn't feel the need to look elsewhere for sexual release.

_____ 36. I believe I couldn't feel any sexier than I do now.

_____ 37. I believe I couldn't be any sexier in my husband's eyes than I am now.

_____ 38. I experience orgasm whenever I choose to.

_____ 39. I enjoy experiencing vaginal (G-spot) orgasms.

_____ 40. I enjoy clitoral orgasms.

_____ 41. I am able to achieve multiple orgasms.

_____ 42. I believe I am a good steward of my sexuality and the power it holds.

_____ 43. I believe my husband is a good steward of his sexuality and the power it holds.

_____ 44. I believe sex bonds me and my husband together in a special and unique way.

_____ 45. I do not struggle with issues of low self-esteem.

_____ 46. I feel worthy of a man's attention and affection.

_____ 47. I do not feel inferior to any other woman.

_____ 48. I am not haunted by sexual "ghosts" in my past.

_____ 49. I do not bear any scars from previous sexual abuse or experiences.

_____ 50. Sexual intimacy does not elicit any negative emotions at all.

_____ 51. I don't worry about what others might think if they knew my sexual past.

_____ 52. I don't fear being drawn toward previous lovers.

_____ 53. I don't fear being drawn toward new extramarital lovers.

_____ 54. I am comfortable with my own sexual fantasies.

_____ 55. I have no problem verbalizing my sexual fantasies to my husband.

_____ 56. I make personal hygiene a daily priority so I never have to worry about unpleasant odors.

_____ 57. My bedroom is a place that provides a sexual sanctuary in my marriage.

_____ 58. I believe I look sexy in the underwear I choose to wear.

_____ 59. I don't believe there is any "morally wrong" sexual position within marriage.

_____ 60. My spirituality and sexuality are not in conflict with each other.

_____ 61. I am willing to be on top in bed if it stimulates my husband to watch me.

_____ 62. I consistently make time for sex because it's an important aspect of our lives.

_____ 63. I believe our sex life is at least "normal" or "better than normal."

_____ 64. My children feel free to ask me about or discuss sexual issues.

_____ 65. I am comfortable initiating conversations with my children about sexuality.

_____ 66. I believe my children want a marriage like mine someday.

_____ 67. I believe my husband sees me as a sexually confident wife.

_____ 68. I see myself as a sexually confident wife.

_____ 69. Based on my example, I believe my daughter will be a sexually confident wife someday.

I'm not going to give you a scale by which you can give yourself a "grade," because it's not about how our numbers average out. It's about celebrating our strengths and being willing to work on our weaknesses. Just glance back over your numbers and you'll recognize the areas in which you have the most confidence and which areas need improvement.

Beyond Competence to Confidence

Most women are sexually *competent*. They know what to do in the bedroom to bring their husband to climax. But I want more than that for you. I want you to be sexually *confident*. Sexual confidence isn't just for the supermodel or porn star. It is the birthright of every woman, and the deep desire of every husband for his wife. It's also a valuable legacy that we pass down to our own daughters and granddaughters as they are seeking to understand, embrace, and celebrate their own sexuality within marriage.

However, issues such as extreme body inhibition, shame from past sexual abuse, guilt over premarital sexual activity, fear of intimacy, or lack of knowledge about male and female sexuality are just some of the many hurdles that hold us back in the bedroom.

If you could overcome all of the hurdles holding you back, could you become a sexually confident wife? Absolutely! If that is your desire, let's figure out how to overcome these hurdles and get on the right track toward sexual confidence.

As I wrote this book, the same question was posed by several well-intentioned, marketing-minded friends: "Why don't you call it *The Sexually Confident Woman* instead of *The Sexually Confident Wife*?" While I appreciated their encouragement to reach a larger audience, the suggestion simply didn't sit right with me.

I'm not so sure that a single woman struggles nearly as much with sexual confidence as married women do. Marriage is intended to be a rich, rewarding relationship that provides a unique bond between a husband and wife, and a lifelong commitment is potentially the greatest source of comfort and strength one could experience in a lifetime. But marriage requires hard work, and the sexual aspect of the relationship is no different. When things become difficult in the bedroom, it can be a real temptation for a wife to withdraw both physically and emotionally rather than putting forth the effort to keep things fresh and exciting.

On the other hand, it's not hard for a single woman to keep sex fresh and new when her relationship *is* fresh and new. She is often wined, dined, and romanced. But the more typical scenario for the married woman is an evening meal of leftovers from the fridge, followed by dinner dishes, writing out bills and balancing the checkbook, helping kids with homework, baths, and bedtime stories, and switching a load of laundry so everyone will have clean clothes to wear the next day. She may crawl into bed exhausted, wondering, *Does he even recognize all I do around here? . . . Does he understand how much I long to feel appreciated and affirmed? . . . Will he understand if I'm simply not in the mood tonight? . . . Does he still think I'm beautiful even with these stretch marks and post-pregnancy pounds? . . . Does he still love me after all these years?*

When a single woman seduces her man, she's a rock star in his eyes. But the married woman can feel more like a falling star. After a decade or three of marriage, she may find it difficult to come up with any technique or position they haven't already tried hundreds of times. She may even feel a deep sense of rebellion rising up to declare, "I don't even like sex anymore!" Or worse, she may be sexually interested, only to have her husband lose interest in her. *Ouch!*

I'd even go so far as to say that a single man and woman aren't even having real sex. They're having "best foot forward" sex (or whatever body part you want to use to describe it). They're showing each other only their good side, then retreating to the safety of their singleness. In marriage, however, there's no retreating. Living in close quarters all these years, we see not just the good but also the bad and the ugly, both in our husbands and in ourselves. We have to learn to arouse and be aroused by each other from day to day, month after month, year after year, in spite of those little idiosyncrasies that can drive us crazy at times.

Indeed, sexual confidence can be a great challenge for a married woman, but I believe this book is going to help you on many different levels—emotionally, mentally, physically, and spiritually. Rather than feeling as if sexual confidence is unrealistically *required* of you as a wife, I hope this book will truly *inspire* it in you.

And if you'd like to inspire other wives with your story, visit our blog page at www.sexuallyconfidentwife.com.

2

Getting on the Right Track

Extra space was hard to come by in my first apartment. My couch, coffee table, and television ate up almost every square inch of my combination living room/kitchenette, and my bedroom was filled wall-to-wall with a queen-size bed, dresser, and two nightstands. With some determination, however, I managed to squeeze a treadmill into the corner of my bedroom near the closet door.

As I came home from work each day, eager to shuck my business suit and panty hose, my treadmill became less and less of a workout machine and more and more of a clothesline. Although my clothes remained relatively clean and wrinkle-free dangling from the hand-rails, my body remained relatively weak and flabby. I'd have been much better off taking the extra five seconds to hang the clothes in the closet, then using the treadmill for a good workout.

Any time we use something for a purpose other than which it was created, we don't get the maximum benefits. I could use my car to store numerous boxes to keep them safe from the weather, but then I'd have no transportation for my family. I could use my laptop as a snack tray, but then I'd never write another book or send another e-mail. It's only by using things according to the purpose for which they were created that we get the most benefit from them.

Our sexuality is very much the same way. We can use sex for a wide variety of reasons. We can manipulate and control our husbands, giving sexual favors as a reward for good behavior or withholding sex as a punishment for bad behavior. We're able to appease our partners, giving in to an occasional quickie just to get his paws off us for a while. Or we can frustrate our husbands, creating expectations in our minds that he can never live up to. But none of these fulfill the purpose of sexual intimacy (although many women are using sex for these very reasons).

Of course, the sexual revolution of the 1960s and seventies taught us that sex was simply about feeling good. "If it feels good, do it!" the bumper stickers read. So many of us did it, and it felt good for a while, but the good feelings didn't last. Younger women are beginning to echo the same sentiment. Many Generation Xers and Yers have found that "hooking up" and having "friends with benefits" hasn't prepared them for a lifetime of marital bliss as much as a lifetime of marital stress. Could all of these sexual freedoms that women now enjoy actually be stunting our growth into mature, sexually confident women? I believe so. We've become so confused about the real purpose of sexuality that we're wandering way off track rather than pursuing genuine intimacy and relational fulfillment. For example,

- Today we have sex toys and vibrators of every size, shape, and color, but do we understand that sex isn't just a game we play to achieve orgasm? Do we understand our most basic needs as sexual beings? Do we know how to get those needs met?
- We have female condoms, morning-after pills, and all sorts of

birth control options, but do we have control over our own sexual identity? Do we know what we really want in order to feel intimately connected to another human being?

- We have pornography at the click of a mouse, steamy love stories on HBO, and wild romance novels on our bookshelves, but are we passionate about our own marriage relationship? Do we know how to keep the home fires burning?

If you aren't sure how to answer these questions, perhaps you need to get on the right track toward sexual fulfillment and discover (or rediscover) the three purposes (or three Ps) of sexuality:

1. Procreation
2. Pleasure
3. Pair-bonding.

The Three Ps of Purposeful Sexuality

Most of us are well aware of the procreation aspect. Those beautiful babies women give birth to? They are created through the act of sex. Hopefully that's no news flash to you, so we won't spend much time on this aspect. The upside of using sex for procreation is that we are able to produce sweet little bundles of joy that closely resemble two unique gene pools and are a constant reminder of our blissful (or once blissful) marital union. Children give us great cause for celebration, and more Kodak moments than we could ever completely capture in the thickest of Creative Memories scrapbooks. The downside, however, is that it can take only one sexual encounter to produce a child. If procreation is the only reason a wife engages in sex, she's going to have one sex-starved relationship.

Which leads us to the next purpose of sexual intimacy: to provide pleasure. Hopefully you've experienced it—that erotic feeling of abandoning all inhibitions and just going with the sexual flow. That supernatural, euphoric feeling of slowly ascending to the highest peak of physical pleasure. That wave of complete satisfaction that suddenly washes over you—a wave that is absolutely impossible to verbalize, regardless of how creative your vocabulary may be. And the overwhelming joy of witnessing your partner's eyes roll back in his head and the guttural sounds emitting from his mouth, indicating that he's going over the top, and it's *you* who is ushering him there. Of all the physical pleasures known to man and woman, none compares with sexual arousal and climax.

However, I believe there is something that sexual intimacy can provide that is even more precious and coveted by women than pretty babies and great orgasms. What might that be? Listen as these women try to explain their deepest desire.

- "My husband wants to look at my body, but what I really want him to see is *me*. Behind these big breasts is a heart yearning for a spiritual connection."
- "I don't care about intercourse. I care about intimacy. If I had to choose between a roll in the sheets or a stroll in the park, I'd pick the park every time."
- "I don't want an all-night sexual marathon, just one hour of his attention and affection."

I'm tempted to send these comments to spammers that send out stupid e-mails like *Take Viagra—she'll love you for it! . . . Ejaculate like a porn star! . . . Add three inches overnight! . . . Fill her mouth completely!* Doesn't anyone get it? A woman isn't as interested in having her tonsils tickled as having her soul touched. Her innermost need is for an emotional and spiritual bond with another human being—a need called "pair-bonding," which is actually the third purpose of sexuality. Every healthy woman longs to feel intimately connected—mind, body, heart, and soul—with her mate.

But for all those women who want the emotional connection *instead of* the physical connection, I have a revolutionary news flash: There is scientific evidence that proves you'd be spinning your wheels to try to get one without the other.

Creating Sexual Balance

The secret to having the marriage of your dreams is understanding the need for "sexual balance" in the relationship. To help you understand this concept, let's look at what I call the Seesaw of Sexuality. Our sexuality has four unique components: the physical, mental, emotional, and spiritual. Though every individual's psyche is made up of these four components, two seem to be more important to the male soul and the other two weigh heavier with the female soul, creating a seesaw effect that looks something like this:

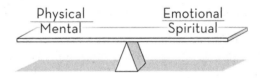

Keeping these components of our sexual relationship in balance is an art form and the goal of the sexually confident wife. If things get out of balance one way or another, either the husband or the wife can feel cheated and used. She can feel like nothing more than a piece of meat because he's getting his physical needs met while she starves emotionally. Or he feels like her little lapdog: she's getting lots of his time and attention, but he gets nothing more than a pat on the head to meet his physical needs.

A sexually confident wife not only will be able to maintain a balance between his needs and her needs, but will also recognize how they all work together to create synergy in the relationship. It's no longer about keeping score or who's getting his or her own way. It's about how the physical, mental, emotional, and spiritual are all combining to form a magical elixir that keeps them both intoxicated with passion for each other.

Understanding Our Sexual Layers

When it comes to marital intimacy for a woman, these four components of sexuality can best be prioritized by visualizing them as multiple layers found beneath the earth's surface, with the physical dimension being the most superficial and the spiritual dimension being the deepest, most fulfilling level of connection.

Again, for a woman, the most superficial of sexual connections is the physical. Don't get me wrong. Sex feels great. But anyone can touch our bodies, and many men seem eager to do so. A mental connection is somewhat more fulfilling, as he sparks our imagination and stimulates us intellectually with deep conversations. An emotional connection is even better, as our heart is stirred and drawn in his direction because of his obvious care and compassion for us. But a spiritual connection is the ultimate sexual experience!

When our husband takes the time to look past the externals of what we look like, to look beyond what we can do for him, and to recognize *who we are* as a beautiful person created in the image of God, that is when we feel valued and cherished. The same is true in how a wife looks at a husband. He wants you to think he's eye candy and he wants you to appreciate all that he does for you, but his greatest desire is for you to respect who he is in the core of his being. This type of pair-bond, coupled with a deep spiritual connection with the Creator of masculinity, femininity, and sexuality, creates indescribable euphoria in the depth of our soul. Even better than a mind-blowing orgasm is a mind-boggling soul-to-soul connection with another human being (which, serendipitously, most often leads to the best mind-blowing orgasms!). When we experience this kind of deep spiritual connection over and over within marriage, it fulfills us in a way that nothing and no one else possibly can.

However, just as we can't get to the innermost layers of the earth without going through the surface, we can't get to the innermost emotional and spiritual layers of our sexuality without first going through the physical and mental. In fact, there's scientific evidence that humans need physical touch to feel fully connected to another human being. I call this scientific evidence "the big O!"—standing not for *orgasm* (which we'll talk more about in Chapter 4) but rather for *oxytocin*.

The "Big O!" Hormone

When we are tenderly touched by another human being, a wonderful hormone called oxytocin is released. Then what happens? We feel good about the person who touched us and we crave even more touch from the same person. It creates a powerful, relationship-building upward spiral. The more we're touched, the more we want to be touched, and the more touching going on, the more oxytocin is being produced. It's like a powerful magnet drawing us together with greater and greater force.

Oxytocin is exponentially more effective when coupled with estrogen (which women produce far more of than men), which explains why women form such a deep emotional bond with their sex partners and have a more difficult time "letting go and moving on" than men do when a relationship crumbles.[1] This also explains why women place far more weight on the "emotional/spiritual" side of sexuality than on the "physical/mental" side. We simply fail to recognize that it's the "physical" side that results in such a strong emotional connection in the first place.

Oxytocin can be triggered by emotional cues such as the glance of a lover or the sound of a loved one's voice. These cues can create stars in our eyes, fireworks in our mind, and swarms of butterflies in our stomach. This hormone increases testosterone production in both men and women, which sends our sex drive into high gear, and oxytocin levels skyrocket to the highest levels when women experience orgasm.[2] As our nipples and genitals are stimulated, even more oxytocin is produced, which creates an overwhelming desire for sexual intercourse and orgasmic response, which creates more oxytocin, and so on, and so on. If you want to reignite the flame of marital passion, oxytocin is just the fuel you need.

So the next time you feel as if you're hitting a sexual wall and you can't imagine "giving in" to his sexual advances, simply determine to climb over that wall instead. You may very well experience what many other sexually confident wives experience on the other side of that wall—absolute euphoria.

"The intimacy in sex is never only physical. In a sexual relationship we may discover who we are in ways otherwise unavailable to us, and at the same time we allow our partner to see and know that individual.
As we unveil our bodies, we also disclose our persons."
—Dr. Thomas Moore,
American theologian, writer

Also be aware that oxytocin production (or the lack thereof) can work against your sex drive. If this hormone isn't being released in your system regularly, you may feel an overwhelming temptation to withdraw emotionally and physically, creating a downward spiral in the relationship. Perhaps you or your husband is not satisfied with how often you experience "the big O" (orgasm) or how often you desire to engage in any sort of sexual activity, but the real culprit may be that you don't get enough of the "big O!" hormone (oxytocin). If a woman isn't touched regularly enough outside the bedroom, she may find that she is violently opposed to being touched inside the bedroom. A vicious cycle is created, as she is no longer open to the very touch she needs.[3] The remedy for not feeling like you want to touch or be touched by your husband, therefore, is to touch anyway. Go through the actions, and your feelings quickly catch up. Oxytocin production ensures this will be the case.

I would never be so cold as to say to a woman struggling with her sexuality, "Get over it, and get naked!" But I'll let you do the math. One naked, oxytocin-producing man plus one naked, oxytocin-producing woman equals one intimately connected couple.

If you need a second opinion, here's what Paul and Lori Byerly (authors of *The Generous Husband* and *The Generous Wife*) have to say:

> The fact that sex increases oxytocin levels can be helpful for women who complain they "never feel like sex." Having sex, even when you don't have a drive to do so, will actually affect you in ways that will result in a greater sex drive. This also explains, at least in part, why many women find that the more sex they have, the more they want, and the less sex they have, the less they want.[4]

Many women mistakenly assume that they only need sex when they are horny. But a woman's horny radar often reads "Zero-Zip-Zilch-Nada." However, that doesn't mean she doesn't need to feel pair-bonded with her husband. In our house, we have numerous kinds of sex rather than just "I'm horny" sex. We have make-up sex to bring closure to disagreements, celebration sex to share joy over an accomplishment, comfort sex when our skies are feeling a little gray, connection sex whenever one of us is about to leave town, and so on.

Maybe you are thinking, *But I'm too stressed out to have sex.* Good news! Oxytocin also serves as a stress reducer. Even just holding hands, playing footsie, or giving/getting a massage releases oxytocin into your system, creating a sense of attachment and the desire to cuddle up close.[5] Not only that, but studies involving both celibate women and sexually active women reveal that oxytocin production (through regular orgasmic experiences) can also help prevent cancer, so sex doesn't just feel good—it's also good for your health![6]

So when you experience even an inkling of those warm, fuzzy feelings, don't pull away or busy yourself with something else. There's nothing more important than feeling this special connection with your special guy. In doing so, you are fulfilling the main purpose of our sexuality—to strongly pair-bond us.

Getting Sticky Again

I wish I had known what a powerful glue oxytocin is much earlier in life. It could have helped me connect more intimately with my husband much earlier in our marriage. It also could have helped prevent me from "pair-bonding" so deeply with many other men beforehand. Little did I know that sexual intimacy is like a clear strip of sticky packing tape, bonding us tightly to each other. When that bond is broken, we lose physical, mental, emotional, and spiritual fragments of our being to that person. We are stuck with similar fragments of the other person, creating "baggage" we carry around internally until we manage to sever those soul ties (which we'll talk about in Chapter 5). It becomes harder and harder to stay connected with another human being because we are so accustomed to breaking that bond over and over such that our "tape" is no longer sticky.

But becoming a sexually confident wife is all about restoring the stickiness of your tape. It's about learning to connect intimately with your husband, not just physically but mentally, emotionally, and spiritually as well. It's about getting on the right track toward genuine intimacy and fulfillment, and rediscovering the true purpose of sexuality—to create a powerful bond between husband and wife that fuels our deepest passions and satisfies our very souls.

Part 2

Confronting Ghosts
from the Past

3

Rewinding Our Childhood Tapes

When I was a girl, my mom used to tease me that I was going to wear out the Rewind button on my stereo. I couldn't get enough of my favorite songs, such as Elvis Presley's "Burning Love" and Elton John's "Crocodile Rock." Instead of listening to the whole cassette tape and just enjoying my favorite song each time it came around, I'd keep rewinding the tape and playing the song over and over again, sometimes ten or twelve times in a row!

Unfortunately, these weren't the only tapes I was in the habit of rewinding and replaying again and again. I also had mental tapes that I replayed—tapes that reminded me of all my negative attributes, tapes that brainwashed me into believing things like these:

I'm unworthy of living.
No one wants to be around me because I'm ugly.
I don't deserve a man's love.

As a mature adult woman, I now recognize these thoughts as complete lies that robbed me of my confidence for too many years.

However, when I was younger, I couldn't always discern the differ-ence between the truth and a lie, and I usually found the lies much easier to believe. I think most women do something similar—we latch on to random lies about who we are, and we allow these lies to negatively affect our self-esteem and rob us of our confidence in life. And does that have an impact on our sexual confidence? You bet it does.

Tracing Our Negative Mental Tapes

It is often helpful to trace certain lies back to their origin so we can recognize where they came from and how they got started in our minds. Then it is easier to realize their falsehood and re-record new mental tapes—tapes that reflect the truth about who we really are. To illustrate this beneficial exercise, we'll use the three examples I just gave.

Lie #1:
I'm not worthy of living.

How could such a negative thought invade a young mind? For me, it came as a result of a very traumatic experience deeply rooted in my childhood memory bank. The first four years of my life were spent basking in the presence of my adoring big sister, Donna. We also had an older brother, Bill, but he was usually out doing boy stuff while Donna and I played countless hours with our dolls, tea party set, and old maid cards.

One hot summer day in 1972, eight-year-old Donna complained of a headache, and later began vomiting uncontrollably. I was only four years old at the time, but I remember it all vividly. I was sent to a neighbor's house and Donna was whisked away to the emergency room. When I returned home the next day, every room of our house was filled with people and the air was filled with the scent of Kentucky Fried Chicken. My mother was passed out on the couch with people fanning her, and my dad was sobbing in his bed. As I climbed into his arms, he wailed, "Sissy's dead. She's never coming back." I didn't know what "dead" meant, but I knew what "never coming back" meant, and I wondered if I was somehow to blame. I tiptoed into my brother's room, where he was also crying on his bed. I hid behind a chalkboard standing on an easel, partially because I feared it would embarrass my brother to be seen crying, and partially because I wanted to disappear and come back another day to find that today had just been a bad dream.

Several years later, I overheard my mother joking with a friend, saying, "We had already sold the crib when we heard Shannon was coming!" I put two and two together in my mind. Bill was on purpose. Donna was on purpose. But Shannon was an accident. This exacerbated the notion that *I should have been the one that died,* not Donna. Therefore, the feeling I carried in my spirit throughout childhood and even into adulthood could best be summed up with the words "I'm not worthy of living."

How does this feeling affect a person's sexual self-confidence? If you don't feel you deserve to exist, you don't feel that you deserve happiness, or relational fulfillment, or sexual pleasure. You feel guilty about experiencing anything positive in life, because after all, you really shouldn't even be on the planet in the first place. You feel as if there's only so much good to go around and if anything good happens to you, it must mean you are robbing it from someone else who does deserve it.

Perhaps you've never experienced the loss of such a close loved one, but it may sound familiar to feel undeserving of good things, or even to feel undeserving of life itself. If this feeling rings a bell in your spirit at all, it's time to erase the "I'm not worthy of living" tape and record a new, more truthful message.

The Truth:
Every person has a right to a fulfilling life.

As an adult, I've come to realize that I'm not in control of deciding who lives and who dies. One who has far greater power than I placed me on earth for a reason, and He took my sister for a reason. I don't have to fully understand these reasons to accept that God is in control of life-and-death issues, not me.

And because God has given me life, I have a right to live it, and live it to the fullest. My sister's death does not negate my reason for living. Donna wouldn't have wanted me to die spiritually just because she died physically. She wouldn't want me to feel forever guilty about existing beyond her death, as if I should have experienced her fate simply because I was the "unplanned one." She would have wanted me to find purpose in going on through life without her, and I've learned to do just that. I can feel sad about her absence, but I don't have to feel unworthy of life. There's plenty of good to go around to everyone, so I don't have to feel bad when good things happen to me. I deserve to be happy. I deserve fulfilling relationships, and I deserve to experience sexual pleasure. It's my birthright as a sexual human being.

It's your birthright as well. Perhaps your reasons for feeling unworthy of a fulfilling life differ from mine. Perhaps a childhood bully, or mean-spirited sibling, or even a parent communicated to you somehow that you don't deserve to exist. Remember that it's hurting people who hurt people, so most likely they were projecting their own painful feelings of unworthiness onto you. Don't accept that bag of negativity. Refuse to hold on to any feelings of unworthiness at all. If you're here on the planet, there's a reason. Discover that reason, and live the fulfilling life God intends for you.

Lie #2:
No one wants to be around me because I'm ugly.

Perhaps you've heard this tape replay in your mind over and over again as well. Every girl has to sail some stormy seas on her way through puberty. Some have a rougher ride than others. Although my childhood was much smoother than those of some other women I've counseled, it was bumpy enough to create some deep bruises on my ego.

My first "ugly" feeling came innocently enough from my older brother. He and his friends liked to play around the creek at Cardboard Hill shirtless and in cutoff shorts. As a six-year-old tomboy, I was desperate to fit in with the guys, especially since I'd lost my female playmate when Donna died. So I tried to do everything the boys did, including hanging out at Cardboard Hill in nothing but cutoff shorts. Of course, my twelve-year-old brother went home complaining, "Mom, my friends don't want to see my little sister running around without her shirt on! Tell her that's nasty!" In my six-year-old mind, what I heard my brother saying was "We don't want to look at you because *you* are nasty! You're ugly! Put your shirt back on, or better yet, just go away! Get out of our sight!"

In the coming years, I tried everything to look prettier. I thought my forehead was way too big, so I cut my hair and created bangs to cover it. But then my bangs would never lie right because of the cowlicks along my hairline. I had way too many freckles, so I'd lie in the summer sun trying to get a dark enough tan so that they'd all blend in, not realizing that being in the sun is part of what causes freckles in the first place. Beauty seemed an impossible pursuit, and confidence continually eluded me.

As I was going through puberty, my brother took a picture of me lying on the floor with an open-mouthed grin that showed my buck teeth protruding slightly through my lips. When the picture came back from the photo lab, he laughed, saying I looked like a walrus. That name stuck for several years. Hoping to change my walruslike appearance, I tried dieting off and on as my willpower allowed, and I even wore a rubber band around my buck teeth at night, hoping it would have the same effect as braces, which I knew my parents couldn't afford. Even as my body changed shape and my teeth naturally straightened on their own, I still subconsciously wore the "WALRUS" name tag for many years. Over and over the suspicion resounded in my mind. *No one will ever want to be around me because I'm ugly.* Again, time to record a new, more accurate message.

"When I look in the mirror I see the girl I was when I was growing up, with braces, crooked teeth, a baby face, and a skinny body."
—*Heather Locklear, actress*

The Truth:
People are more naturally drawn to secure, confident women than they are to beauty queens.

We've heard it said that beauty is only skin deep, and that's true when you are dealing with a one-dimensional photograph of a person. Perhaps that magazine model looks great on glossy paper, but getting to know her personally may reveal that she's not a very beautiful person at all. In fact, some of the most externally beautiful women can turn out to be some of the most internally unattractive individuals you'd ever encounter. The truth is that when we are dealing with a three-dimensional image (a real person), beauty isn't just measured by the skin that person is in. It's measured by how she obviously feels about being in that skin.

For example, I have two very different women who are a part of my world. One closely resembles the stereotype of what most women only wish they could look like—gracefully tall with flat abs, slight hips, full breasts, platinum blond hair cascading almost to her buttocks, and flawless bronze skin (I'll call her Lori). At a size four, she could easily pass for Barbie's twin sister. The other woman (whom I'll call Kristie) is more like a size fourteen, with dark brown hair and ivory skin that reveals a scar down the middle of her chest where she had heart surgery as a child. If you ask which of these women a man would ultimately prefer to spend time with once he got to know them, I'd say Kristie would win that toss. If you ask me who has the greater potential for being a sexually confident wife, I'd again say Kristie. As a matter of fact, if you asked me who I'd rather *be* given the choice, I'd say Kristie, hands down. Why? Because of the beauty (or lack thereof) that I see on the *inside* of these women.

Although Lori could pass for a *Playboy* centerfold, she's constantly obsessing over her weight, her posture, her skin, her hair, her makeup, and her clothes. Sure, it's good that a woman takes care of herself, but you can't have a two-minute conversation with Lori without her dredging up her insecurities and fishing for affirmation. It's exhausting. Most women are intimidated by her, and men say they find it difficult to talk to her, probably because it's hard to look Lori in the eye when her shirts so dramatically showcase her breast implants. Therefore, although stunning, Lori is a lonely, miserable woman.

Kristie on the other hand may not have photographers beating down her door, but she is one of the most beautiful and socially secure women I've ever met. She's stunning, but in a completely different way. She couldn't care less what other people think about the size of her thighs or the style of her hair. She's much deeper than that. She's more concerned with how she can help others and make a difference in people's lives. She naturally draws people closer to her, and the closer you get to Kristie, the more her beauty strikes you.

Lori's looks may be superficially enviable, but you couldn't pay me to live in her skin if all of her insecurities come with it. Why? Because people are more naturally drawn to secure, confident women than they are to beauty queens. So ignore the "I'm ugly" tapes and give up the beauty queen dreams. Instead, focus on real beauty—beauty that comes from being happy with the skin you're in, flaws and all.

Lie #3:
I'm not worthy of a man's love.

In my earliest childhood years, I remember being the star of the show. The baby of the family usually gets most of the attention and affection. But when my sister died, it seemed like my star status died with her. Why? Because my family's way of coping with grief seemed to be withdrawal, and a star with no audience no longer feels like a star. Dad withdrew to his workshop most evenings and throughout every weekend I can remember. Bill withdrew to his bedroom, taking solace in his eight-track tapes and headphones. Mom was more available than anyone else, yet the kitchen seemed to be her preferred place of refuge, and learning to cook was never high on my priority list. So I was usually in the living room, wondering, *Hey! What about me?*

Six years separated me and my brother, and we were never really friends until we were both adults. I remember begging him to take me cruising down Wesley Street in his midnight blue Grand Prix, but he insisted that I crawl down into the floorboard and duck my head down low so that no one saw me. He was most likely thinking, *It wouldn't be cool to be seen with my little sister.* I was thinking, *There must be something wrong with me if he's ashamed to be seen with me.*

I think I understood that this kind of relationship was pretty par for the course between big brothers and their little sisters, but I couldn't understand why Dad was so much more interested in what he had going on in his shop than in what was going on in my life. He was always too busy to attend my special functions. I have absolutely no recollection of my dad ever attending a single choir recital, drama or pep squad performance, awards ceremony, or church service. It was always just me and Mom going by ourselves. With the overt withdrawal of every important male in my life, it could only stand to reason in my young mind that *I was not worthy of a man's love, time, or attention.* But my big-girl mind has memorized a new message . . .

The Truth:
I have much to offer and am worthy of healthy relationships.

Even though my relationships with my father and brother have grown much closer since I've become an adult, as a child I always thought I was missing out. I was envious of my friends whose dads were always in the audience, cheering them on and beaming proudly as they bragged about their daughters' talents. I saw siblings hanging out together at the mall and enjoying each other's company, and

I felt so alone. However, I wasn't the only one missing out. My dad and brother were robbing themselves as well.

The truth is that if others fail to see what a valuable person you are, it's their loss. Their lack of interest doesn't decrease your value. It simply takes away from the fulfillment they could ultimately experience in life by knowing you more intimately. But when this disinterest comes from a significant male in your childhood, it's hard not to replay the "I'm not worthy" message over and over in our minds.

How do we rewind that tape and record a new message? It was a two-step process for me. First, I had to realize that my dad's emotional unavailability had nothing to do with me. It was his own issue. Again, it's hurting people who hurt people, and the reason my father hurt me so deeply was because he was hurt so deeply as a child yet never sought healing for those wounds. His parents divorced when he was a young boy, and they frequently sent him back and forth from one home to the next. Neither parents nor step-parents seemed to want to raise him or spend time with him. After being verbally and physically abused, he left home as a young teenager. His grandparents took him in, but he carried these wounds of rejection into adulthood, nursing them the only way he knew how—by remaining busy, distracted, and withdrawn.

How could I choose to forgive him? It was my way of trying to show him the unconditional love he never received as a child. I knew I'd fare much better in life if I didn't hold a grudge against him, and I was determined not to repeat the exact pattern with my children by walking around wounded. Forgiveness was the only way of drawing a line in the generational sand and declaring, "The dysfunction stops with me. The healing starts now." Of course, every family has to deal with a certain amount of dysfunction, but I've tried to put the *fun* back in dys*fun*ctional, hoping my children would have an easier time of coping with their own childhood issues as I eagerly try to cope with my own.

The second step to recording a new "I am worthy!" tape was to basically "reparent" myself for a season. I could mourn all of the things I missed out on as a girl, or I could re-create opportunities to fill my own "worthiness" cup. Instead of being angry that Dad failed to invest time or energy in taking me places or doing things with me, I decided to do them for myself. I took myself to the zoo and fed the animals. I took myself to the movies and ate the whole bucket of popcorn. I went for walks at the Dallas Arboretum, smelling all of my favorite flowers. I took myself out to lunch at my favorite restaurants. I bought myself a pretty scarf, or a gourmet chocolate truffle, or a new CD. I listened to music and danced alone in my living room. I enjoyed myself without inhibition. And I felt sorry for the men in my life that had never learned to enjoy these simple pleasures with me.

What effect did this have on my marriage and sex life? I was no longer angry with my husband for not filling the void left by my father and brother. These experiences helped me take the weight of responsibility off his shoulders to be my emotional all-in-all. Any attention and affection Greg gave me became just an extra layer of icing on my cake. And our sex life thrived, because not only did I feel love for the man I was with but I also felt love for myself, which doubled my passion quotient.

Reshaping Our Sexuality

Perhaps you never made the connection between the negative messages embedded into your brain as a child and the inhibition you feel in the bedroom as a grown woman. Indeed, our sexuality is shaped by the world we live in, but more important, by the home we grew up in.

Our fathers communicated to us through words and actions (or lack thereof) whether or not we are worthy of the time, attention, and affections of a man. Our mothers communicated to us how we are supposed to behave and interact as women of worth and value. But so often that baton of confidence never gets passed. Why? Because parents can't give what they don't have. If their emotional tank was empty, you probably felt rather empty as well.

These childhood feelings of worthiness or worthlessness spill over into our marriage and family relationships. We often expect our husband to fill the cavernous void left by an emotionally unavailable father, or we look to our daughters for the connection and fellowship we missed out on with our mothers, sometimes smothering them in the process. Rather than grow impatient with everyone else for not satisfying your emotional needs, learn to satisfy them yourself. As an adult woman, you can't expect self-confidence to be bestowed upon you by anyone else. It now has to come from within. Learn to give yourself the gift of self-acceptance. Give yourself the gift of unconditional love. Laud attention and affection on yourself by treating yourself gently and with special care.

Most important, rewind those old mental tapes. Erase them if necessary, and record new affirming messages that you deserve to live, love, be loved, and to be happy with yourself.

4

Healing the Scars of Sexual Abuse

'd just celebrated my thirteenth birthday, and I slipped on my new
pastel striped sweater in anticipation of everyone's arrival. It was
the Sunday before Christmas in 1980, and lots of aunts, uncles,
cousins, and grandparents were due to arrive to celebrate the Christmas holidays, just like we did every year.

My mom was in the kitchen making deviled eggs and babysit-
ting the glazed ham in the oven. My dad and brother were outside
tinkering underneath a car. I was seated at my vanity table in my
bedroom, putting on the makeup I had finally convinced Mom I was
old enough to wear, and styling my "wings" (Farrah Fawcett–style
bangs). Sitting in front of the mirror, I had my back to my closet
door. It was a pass-through closet that connected my bedroom to my
parents' room. As I was running my brush through my long hair, I
heard the closet door hinges creak slightly. I sensed I wasn't alone in
my room anymore. I looked into the vanity mirror and was startled to
see someone peeking through the crack. Walking over to the closet, I
assumed I'd find my brother playing a prank on me, perhaps imitat-

ing Jack Nicholson in *The Shining*. I was relieved to discover that it was only Uncle Bradley, my step-aunt's husband. Knowing he'd been found out, he opened the door farther and insisted, "I didn't mean to scare you! I just wanted to see how beautiful of a woman you are becoming." In hindsight, the fact that my thirty-something-year-old uncle sneaked into my parents' room, passed through the closet, and was spying on me should have scared the bajeebees out of me. Unfortunately, it didn't.

When it was time to open presents, Uncle Bradley presented me with two small packages wrapped in festive red paper with shimmery gold bows. "Open this one first!" he instructed. It was a roll of Kodak film. *But I don't have a camera,* I thought to myself. Then I realized what must be in the second package, and I got as giddy over opening it as Uncle Bradley was about giving it to me. "It's a camera!" I squealed. I carefully loaded the film inside, and my uncle grabbed me by the hand and escorted me outside onto the front lawn, where he snapped the first set of pictures, encouraging me to "pose pretty" for the camera. For the first time, I felt as if someone was really looking at me. I felt like a princess.

On a future visit, Uncle Bradley invited me into his shiny pickup truck, saying my mom needed some things from town to make dinner. Happy to accompany him, I hopped in, wearing a T-shirt, shorts, and flip-flops. We chitchatted about the family and how school was going. Then Uncle Bradley asked, "So, Shannon . . . how far have you ever gone with a boy?"

"Far enough!" I jokingly replied. At thirteen years old, I had actually never gone beyond kissing a neighbor boy in the back of the school bus (and only because we were dared to). But for some reason, my uncle's question made me feel as if I should be more experienced than that.

"Well, how far would you let *me* go?" he inquired, caressing my bare thigh with his fingertips and grinning slyly.

"We'll just have to see about that someday," I replied awkwardly. Of course, this conversation was to be our little secret, Uncle Bradley said, explaining, "Your parents would never understand our special love for each other."

The flirtatious bantering went back and forth for a couple of years, not just with Uncle Bradley, but also with Uncle Sonny, another step-aunt's husband. While I was staying with my cousin Kay one weekend the spring of my eighth grade year, Uncle Sonny entered the bedroom where we slept. He shook me gently, saying, "Come out here so we don't wake Kay up!"

I shuffled into the hallway in my shortie nightgown, only half awake. Sonny wrapped his arms around me, saying he couldn't sleep. He quietly moaned, "I've been thinking of you all night, and I just had to see what you feel like"—rubbing his hands all over my backside—"and what you taste like!" He kissed my neck and shoulders. My heart broke for my aunt, sleeping soundly in her bed. I didn't have the heart to let her know what her new husband was up to in the living room. When I showed few signs of protest, Sonny pressed his lips hard against mine, forcing his tongue into my mouth and waving it wildly, his coarse mustache bristling against the tender skin of my upper lip, and his cigarette breath almost making me gag. This would be the price I'd have to pay any time I wanted to spend time at my cousin's house. Each time Uncle Sonny drove me home, he'd beg me to let him "stick it in, just for a minute" (no longer referring to his tongue, of course). The thought of having his penis inside me repulsed me to the core. I didn't have a hard time refusing his requests.

But Uncle Bradley was a different story. I'd known him all my life, and I'd always thought he was the handsomest man I'd ever laid eyes on. He'd groomed me well with all of his winks, smiles, and sweet nothings whispered when we were out of eyesight and earshot of everyone else. Late one summer morning just before my ninth grade year, Uncle Bradley called, saying he was driving through town. My heart began pounding wildly. "Are your parents at home?" he asked.

"No, they are at work all day. I'm here by myself," I replied.

"Can I come by in about fifteen minutes?"

I responded positively, hung up the phone, and frantically tried to ready myself for his arrival. I brushed my hair and my teeth, shaved my legs, and donned my sexiest satin robe. As I sat on the couch next to Uncle Bradley, he playfully tugged at the hem of my robe, inquiring, "Whatcha got under there?"

"Nothing. You wanna see?" I asked, leading him by the hand to my parents' bedroom. I draped myself across their king-size bed, allowing my robe to fall open. I was exhausted from fighting men like Sonny and other boys off me. At almost fifteen, I thought I was ready to invite one to be my lover. Uncle Bradley seemed the obvious choice, since he made me feel so special.

However, Bradley hesitated. He stood at the foot of the bed, staring at my almost grown-up body, yet obviously recognizing that I was still a child. He said in a low voice, "I'm sorry. I just can't do this to your parents." He left the house abruptly, and divorced my aunt shortly thereafter. I never saw him again. With Uncle Sonny's marriage also dissolving soon thereafter, I was finally free from their sexual harassment. But this last scene ensured that I'd never tell my parents or anyone else about it. Instead of a victim, I now felt more like a vixen. Deep down, a part of me had come to enjoy all of the attention they showered upon me, even if it had been inappropriate attention. In fact, after Uncle Bradley ran out of the house without touching me, I went to the mall that evening on a subconscious mission. I found a guy who was willing to pay attention to me all evening, and when the mall closed we went to an abandoned house and had sex, which was my way of medicating the emotional pain of Uncle Bradley's rejection.

Some of us are manipulated into believing that we really want to have sex, when all we really want is the attention and affection of an admiring male. Other women may be abused in far more violent ways, such as having sex forced upon them without their consent, sometimes by a stranger, and sometimes by a trusted acquaintance. These experiences often wreak havoc in a person's life and marriage relationship. Here are a few examples.

- In a counseling session, Lynn cries hysterically about how her own father, an ordained minister, used to drive her to the church late at night and grope her in the parking lot, sometimes masturbating himself, other times penetrating her orally, vaginally, anally. He would often begin his ritualistic abuse of his own daughter by insisting, "Lynn, you'd better pray to God that He'll stop me! Pray He'll rescue you!" Of course, when she wasn't rescued, she grew to hate both God and her father, who died shortly before Lynn graduated from high school. Hoping to put all of that behind her, Lynn married a wonderful guy she met in college, but after five years, she divorced him because she simply couldn't embrace the idea of committing the same sexual acts that wounded her so deeply. She now resides with a lesbian woman, although she says their relationship is platonic.
- After seven years of sexual abuse by her stepfather, Rita initiated her first consensual sexual experience at fifteen years old. Fast forward thirty years, five husbands, three children, and four

abortions later, and the idea of initiating sex with her husband feels like an overwhelming challenge. "I've always viewed sex as emotionless. I can respond to his advances by going through the motions, but mustering emotion during sex is an art form that I've not yet mastered."

- Emily e-mails: "When I was a barely a teenager, I often babysat for some close family friends. The husband would drive me home while his wife stayed with the children. One night when I was getting out of the car and hugging him goodbye, he swept his hand across my breast and kissed me, forcing his tongue into my mouth. I cried myself to sleep that night, but told no one. Each time he took me home, he'd take a detour down a dirt road and things progressed further and further, even though I tried fighting him off. One night he managed to get my skirt up and forced his face between my legs, pushing my panties aside enough to begin licking me. Why I didn't scream or run, I'm not sure, but I eventually stopped fighting because, in all honesty, I'd never felt anything so good. Although I refused to let him penetrate me for the first several months, I eventually acquiesced and gave my virginity to a married man. I couldn't understand how I could enjoy being sexually abused, but there was certainly an element of pleasure to being pursued and touched this way. However, now as a married woman, every time my husband and I have sex, I struggle with flashbacks of these encounters and feel guilty all over again. For this reason, I usually try to avoid sex altogether because I don't want to go back down that dirt road in my mind. Will I ever be able to enjoy a normal sexual relationship with my husband?"

- In a letter addressed to me and my husband in response to reading our book *Every Woman's Marriage,* Jim writes about his wife of seventeen years: "Holly was abandoned by her father at birth, sexually abused as a child, date-raped as a teenager, and repeatedly used by men her whole life because of her extraordinary beauty. She is bulimic and clinically depressed. She loathes herself because of all that's happened to her. She doubts anyone's love for her, especially God's and mine. She considers herself unworthy of love, yet her need to feel wanted and desired by a man has led her into a third extramarital affair. I can forgive her for the affairs because I know it's not about me. It's about the enormous pain she's lived her whole life in. How can I help my wife heal from the scars of sexual abuse?"

With approximately one-third of women experiencing some sort of sexual abuse in their lifetime, it's a question many of us wrestle with: *How can we heal the scars of sexual abuse?* Our bodies naturally heal from physical wounds given time, but how can we heal emotional wounds? Although we may have experienced physical pain, sexual abuse is ultimately an offensive attack on our dignity, self-esteem, and sense of sexuality. And what effects do such abuses have on our lives? The most common symptoms of sexual abuse are

- avoiding or being afraid of sex
- approaching sex as an obligation
- experiencing negative feelings such as anger, disgust, or guilt with touch
- having difficulty becoming aroused or feeling sexual sensation
- feeling emotionally distant or not present during sex
- experiencing intrusive or disturbing sexual thoughts and images
- engaging in compulsive or inappropriate sexual behaviors

- experiencing difficulty establishing or maintaining an intimate relationship
- experiencing vaginal pain or orgasmic difficulties[1]

Perhaps some of these symptoms have been an issue for you and you never connected them to your previous sexually abusive experiences. Whether these are new revelations or old news, let's consider how we can reclaim those precious parts of who we are as healthy sexual beings. Entire books have been written on this topic, so I'm not going to pretend that one chapter will suffice and completely heal you of all your past hurts. However, I hope these ten steps toward healing will get you thinking and moving in a healthy direction as you seek to overcome the negative effects that sexual abuse can have on our life and relationships.

Survival Secrets

You may be reading the examples in this chapter and thinking, *That's nothing compared to what I have lived through!* It's terribly sad that in our society, so many women suffer horrific sexual abuse or violent rape, often at the hands of very trusted individuals such as relatives or spiritual leaders. If this has been your experience, I urge you to connect with not only a professional counselor but also a support group for survivors of sexual abuse. Inquire with local counseling agencies, women's shelters, or churches for possible leads on finding such a group.

If this sounds scary to you, remember that we are wounded in relationships with unsafe people, but healing can be found in relationships with safe people—those who've lived through similar experiences and are willing to share their recipes for survival. Not only can we glean from others' experiences, but we can be a tremendous encouragement to them as we share nuggets of wisdom and truth found along the path of our own journey toward healing. ●

<hr>

TEN STEPS TOWARD HEALING FROM SEXUAL ABUSE

1. Assign responsibility and let go of shame.

Regardless of how a girl dresses, walks, or talks, she never deserves or asks to be sexually abused. Every person has the right to say no at any point in an encounter, and when a man doesn't take no for an answer, he's guilty of sexual abuse. Period. Or perhaps you're carrying a sense of shame because you didn't say no, because you were either too young, naive, or inexperienced to assert yourself. But it's never, never, never a child's responsibility to tell an adult to stop abusing her. The responsibility to do the right thing rests solely on the adult, even if the child is parading herself naked in front of him and begging to be sexually touched somehow. The reason we often feel shame over our own abuse is because our perpetrators usually refuse to accept their own guilt or take responsibility for their actions. We know that our abuser should feel shame over his misdeeds, but when he doesn't exhibit shame by asking for forgiveness, that shame becomes a hot potato tossed in our direction and we subconsciously hold on to it. We're made to feel as if we "wanted it" or "asked for it" somehow. Nonsense. Neither guilt nor shame belongs in your court. Place the responsibility solely where it belongs—on the perpetrator— and let go of your sexual shame.

2. Look at your labels, and create new ones if necessary.

When our first experiences with sex involve such negative feelings, we often grow to view sex as "bad," "dirty," "nasty," and so on. And if we experience any natural desire for sex, we consider *ourselves* "bad," "dirty," or "nasty." Nothing could be further from the truth. Consensual sex between two adults who love each other and are committed to one another's well-being is one of the most beautiful and fulfilling experiences imaginable. And when you experience sexual desire, you're nothing short of completely healthy and fully human, since we're all sexual beings by design.

3. Understand who you really are, apart from any abuse.

The word *abuse* can best be understood by breaking it down into syllables: *ab-use* or *ab(normal)-use.* In other words, to abuse something means to use it for a reason other than its intended purpose. When you were abused, you were used for something other than for what you were intended. You, as a healthy female, were intended to someday experience and enjoy a healthy sense of sexuality. Don't let someone else's gross error become your own. Don't continually look at yourself through the lens that your abuser once looked at you through. Remember who you are, and know that someone else's misusing you to satisfy his own selfishness doesn't negate or change who you really are as a valuable human being who is worthy of love and deserving of sexual pleasure.

4. Be honest with your husband about your experiences and feelings.

For a long time, I never told my husband about my uncles' inappropriate conduct or my compliance, fearing he'd view me as "damaged goods" and not want me anymore. However, he knew for years that something had to be holding me back, and he was actually relieved to learn that my hesitations were caused more by past memories than by current issues in our marriage. He was very kind and compassionate, and paid for months of counseling to help me process what had happened in my childhood and how it had affected me. In fact, as I described my disgust with Uncle

Sonny's mustache and cigarette breath, Greg asked, "Is that why you get so angry when someone around you is smoking? And is that why you haven't kissed me nearly as much since I grew a mustache?" I'd never put two and two together, but now that he was doing that math, I couldn't deny the logic. Early the next morning, Greg shaved his mustache completely and we caught up on months of missed kisses. Although our husbands may not have the professional skills to counsel us through the healing process (leave that to the professionals), they can be very supportive if given the opportunity.

5. **Give yourself permission to seek the time and space to heal.**

As married women, we assume that we've signed up to be sexual outlets for life. Sex is simply a wife's duty, right? But chances are, your husband doesn't expect you to be just a sexual vending machine. He wants to connect with not just your body but also your heart, mind, and soul during lovemaking. He wants you to be present and enjoy the encounter, and he's most likely willing to give you what you need in order to get there. As I was going through counseling and learning to reestablish sexual boundaries that had been broken down by my previous abusers, I asked my husband if he could give me a short season where sex was simply not an expectation. He was supportive and asked how long I needed. I asked for two months. However, it only took two weeks before I was clamoring for sex with him. Why? Because I felt so emotionally, mentally, and spiritually affirmed when he offered me the time and space I needed.

6. **Experiment to discover what intimate acts you do feel comfortable with.**

Just because you want to refrain from intercourse for a season doesn't mean you can't enjoy intimate encounters and healthy physical touch. During my supposed two-month sexual sabbatical,

I followed my counselor's advice and experimented with things I did feel comfortable with. I felt comfortable lying in bed together. I felt comfortable being naked in my husband's presence. I felt comfortable having Greg caress my arm, face, back, or thighs. I was comfortable with him masturbating in my presence, but I didn't want to be expected to perform sexually at all. However, as I allowed myself to experience these "safe" activities, my sexual appetite was very quickly reawakened, and the thought of waiting two months to have sex with this wonderful man who loved me so much seemed impossible. Neither of us cried over this boundary being broken, and neither did my counselor! Let your husband know what you are comfortable with. Go only where you feel safe, and don't try to rush the process. But don't be surprised if as your safety zone increases you find yourself desiring and enjoying sexual activities that you once felt threatened by.

7. **Exercise your right to choose when and how you are touched.**

The only way your sexual safety zone can increase is if you know you have the freedom to exercise your personal boundaries. But sometimes it's difficult to find the voice or the words to say, "I'm having a hard time right now!" when we're not used to having that freedom. Therefore, create a signal that says, "I need you to stop." A good signal needs to be both unoffensive and obvious, such as a tight squeeze of his elbow. Explain to your husband that this need to stop has nothing to do with him and everything to do with you trying to feel safe and secure in his arms.

8. **Feel the feelings and let them out in a safe environment.**

There may be times when a sexual abuse survivor experiences overwhelming emotions that she simply doesn't know what to do with. However, repressed emotions create enormous amounts of pent-up anger and can produce deep depression. Rather than take your negative emotions out on your husband (remember, he's your lover, not your abuser), vent them in a safe environment. My safe place was group counseling meetings, where I was able to unapologetically express my anger by tearing up old phone books and pillows, screaming at empty chairs, and writing honest letters to my abusers that I never intended to send. By the time I went home, I was too emotionally exhausted to pick a fight with my husband, which was a good thing.

9. **Break the cycle of abuse.**

Because sexual abuse is an attack on our sexual identity, we often search for restoration in the same places where that identity was originally stolen—in sexually abusive relationships. It's as if we're trying to recreate similar scenarios and power struggles in order to "win" this time. But you'll never win at that game. You'll only continue to hurt yourself and others in the process. Every dysfunctional encounter will add to your sense of sexual shame and confusion and drive you one step closer to insanity as you continue doing the same thing over and over, expecting different results. So instead of running toward an extramarital relationship to help you survive your emotional aches and pains, try a more effective approach. Run toward a counselor who can help you heal, and run toward a more intimate relationship with your husband. Then you can not just survive but thrive in spite of the sexual abuse in your past.

10. **Connect to your spiritual self to foster spiritual healing.**

Again, our bodies naturally heal themselves, but our spirits require a more intentional effort. Although it's our bodies that were attacked, it's ultimately our spirits that feel the most pain and suffer the most consequences. Nurture your spiritual self through prayer, meditation, or worship. Listen to music that calms you and makes you feel good. Savor a soul-stirring book or movie. Enjoy deep conversations with a female spiritual mentor. Allow your spirit to bring to your consciousness what you really need in order to feel better about yourself and your sexuality. Your spirit has the answers. But you must connect with your spiritual self in order to hear those answers.

In addition to these ten steps, the most important thing that any woman can do is to hold on to hope—hope that even a sexual abuse survivor can become a sexually confident, sexually satisfied wife. Carol Tuttle, author of the book *Remembering Wholeness: A Personal Handbook for Thriving in the Twenty-first Century* and the best-selling CD *Healing Sexual Abuse and Sexual Issues in Marriage,* writes:

> Having a healthy sexual experience was almost impossible for me the first fifteen years of my marriage. Ten years into my marriage is when I discovered the deeper issues of sexual abuse that had complicated it so much. I did not know how to stay in my adult presence and feel safe in the experience. I continually felt like I was being abused all over again as I had as a child.
>
> To help me heal this, I created an imagery . . . before I would have sex with my husband I would call in my "little Carols" and meet with them and explain that I was choosing to have sex with my husband and it did not involve them. They were not a part of it. I brought in a guardian angel to take them away to a safe place far enough removed from my experience, where they could play and be free.
>
> I would have images of these "little Carols" jumping for joy, saying to me, "Good, we don't want anything to do with that stuff!" I used this technique repeatedly and as a result, I gained

more and more presence as an adult woman who wanted to enjoy sex with her husband . . .

I am a free woman enjoying sex several times a week.[2]

Carol is a free woman. I am a free woman. We know lots of other free women, and you can be free, too—free from the painful scars that disfigure your soul, free of the weight that so easily weighs a woman down, free to experience and enjoy healthy intimacy in a safe relationship—free to be a sexually confident wife!

5

Cutting Soul Ties That Bind

Greg and I were walking through the downtown streets of a quaint little bed-and-breakfast town one Saturday morning in the spring of 1998. We'd stolen away to look at some hard questions, particularly "Why is Shannon so tempted to engage in an emotional affair with yet another inappropriate guy?"

We'd had some gut-wrenching conversations during the eight-hour car ride and throughout the night before. This morning we were taking a break from the mind-numbing mental exercise of trying to figure out what was really going on, just walking hand in hand and soaking up some of the local ambiance.

We wandered into a bookstore on the downtown square and drifted in separate directions. Shortly, Greg approached me with a small book in his hands and asked, "Would you let me buy this for you, as a special gift from me?" It was Robin Norwood's *Daily Meditations for Women Who Love Too Much*. As I thumbed through the cartoon-filled pages, I felt as if that book had been written just for me, just for this season of my life. Greg obviously sensed that as well.

He said he couldn't be mad at me for being such a loving person. He simply wanted me to stop loving other men too much!

One of the most revealing meditations read:

> For clues to your personal style [of loving too much], consider the common themes expressed in your favorite work of fiction, your favorite film, your favorite song, poem, fairy tale, etc. Taken together they will almost certainly provide you with insight into how you go about the business of living and loving—too much.[1]

It didn't take much pondering to figure it out. Favorite fiction novel? *The Scarlet Letter.* Favorite movie? *The Thorn Birds.* Favorite song? Any song from the *Phantom of the Opera* musical soundtrack. Examined together, these works revealed the lessons my soul longed to teach me.

The Scarlet Letter had been the focus of a research paper my senior year of high school. I was fascinated by the story of Hester Prynne, a married woman who (in the long-term absence of her husband) gives in to her passions for her minister, Arthur Dimmesdale. When Hester becomes pregnant with Dimmesdale's child, her growing belly announces to the world that she's committed sexual sin. The townspeople insist that she forever pin a scarlet letter *A* to her clothing as a constant symbol of her adultery. Although her reputation is brought low, Hester keeps her head held high. However, Dimmesdale never comes clean about his part in the adulterous affair. He clings to his sterling reputation while Hester has hers dragged through the dirt. He daily dons his black and white priestly garments while Hester adorns her chest with the harsh red reminder. Dimmesdale's guilty conscience gradually gnaws away at his soul, while Hester ultimately is liberated from the chains of public opinion. Such a scandal stirred me to the core.

Along the same lines, *The Thorn Birds* was a television miniseries that I watched religiously as a teenager, then rented in its entirety many times as an adult. My heart ached for Meggie, a young girl who grows up in an emotionally disconnected family, loses her father and closest brother in an accident, and looks for solace in her close friendship with Father Ralph de Bricassart. As Meggie blossoms into a woman, her fascination with Father Ralph takes on new meaning, as does his fondness for her. Meggie longs to have him in her life, not just as a priest but as a partner. But Father Ralph has his eye on the Vatican, hoping to climb the papal ladder. He spurns her amorous advances, saying, "I do love you, Meggie, but I love God more!" However, fast forward several years, and in a moment of weakness on a remote tropical island, Meggie and Ralph are swept up by their passions and consummate their love for each other. Nine months later, Meggie bears his child and keeps his paternity as secretive as their private rendezvous on that beach. Like Arthur Dimmesdale, Father Ralph hides his guilt with his priestly garments.

I first heard the soundtrack to *The Phantom of the Opera* while riding in my boss's car in my early twenties. She explained the story line about how Christine, a young opera singer, is seemingly possessed by an opera house ghost, who becomes her mentor, or her "angel of music." Although he hides his disfigured face behind a mask, he visits her and lures her into his dark catacombs beneath the opera house, attempting to seduce her into becoming his own. Falling under his spell, Christine feels torn between her beloved musical mentor and Raoul, her childhood sweetheart whose love for her is much more pure and selfless than that of the phantom. But Christine feels supernaturally drawn in the phantom's direction, almost as if their souls are connected somehow. Indeed, she has grown to see him as a father figure since the death of her own father. She feels she has no control over her own life or her own choices, for she is a princesslike pawn in the phantom's musical game.

So what is the common thread between *The Scarlet Letter*, *The Thorn Birds*, and *The Phantom of the Opera?* A woman who loses herself to a man, surrendering her mind, body, or soul (or all three) in hopes of discovering that which her heart yearns for. However, such fulfillment ultimately eludes each one of these women, and in the end she must awaken from her trance and recognize that *he's* not the answer to all of her longings. Hester Prynne deals with the emotional fallout of having given her body to a man who is willing to privately have sex with her but is unwilling to publicly commit his life to her. Meggie learns that she'll always have to take a backseat to God in Father Ralph's heart, and not even her body, heart, and soul on a silver platter will move her to the frontrunner's position. Christine finally gets it when Raoul insists, "Whatever you believe, this man, this thing, is *not* your father!" By the end of the musical, she recognizes that she hasn't been possessed but rather obsessed with the idea of having an angel to lead, guide, and direct her. She declares, "Angel of music, you deceived me! I gave you my mind blindly!"

Yes, it's the hurdle that all women must overcome—the tendency to blindly give ourselves away in the hopes of earning a man's everlasting love. We allow our minds to become obsessed. We allow our bodies to be possessed. We carelessly tie our heartstrings to a man's, creating soul ties that eventually bind us together long after the last goodbye is said. These romantic obsessions, shattered dreams, and bittersweet memories linger, often robbing us of our sexual self-confidence when we realize that he was more of a loser than the ideal lover. We secretly wonder, *If I gave myself to Prince*

Charming and he turned out to be a toad instead, what does that make me? In all honesty, it simply makes us foolish, love-hungry women. But the good news is that we don't have to remain that way. Dysfunctional relationships are not a life sentence. Relational mistakes can equate to valuable lessons learned, and valuable lessons learned can equate to wisdom and confidence.

What valuable lessons did my soul long to teach me as I was reading *The Scarlet Letter,* watching *The Thorn Birds,* and listening to *Phantom of the Opera* music over and over again? Read on, and I think you'll find the answers obvious.

Making a List, Checking It Twice

Shannon: 50+

Greg: 0

That's how the scorecard would have read had there been one. I'd walked into marriage at twenty-two years old with more than fifty sexual partners in my past. Greg, at twenty-six, was still a virgin. Together, we flew in the face of conventional stereotypes of the sexually experienced macho male and the pure-as-the-driven-snow female. As I entered counseling several years into our marriage, my main goals were to get the scarlet letter off my sweater, cut the soul ties that had bound me for too long, and rid my mind of the relational ghosts that continued to haunt me.

My counselor's challenge was simple enough. Make a list of all your sexual partners and figure out what all of them have in common. Sounds easy, right? Not if your scorecard is as full as mine. It took several weeks, and the floodgates of emotion burst wide open as I began digging for answers to the question "And *why* did I sleep with *him?*" over and over. However, a distinct pattern soon surfaced. More than 95 percent of these men had been older than I was, and most had had some type of authority over me. Translation: Just like Hester, Meggie, and Christine, I'd been blindly giving myself away, hoping to find a loving father figure to help me feel safe, secure, and special. But my tactics had backfired royally. My lifestyle had become very dangerous, creating major insecurities and robbing me of any notion that I was or could ever be special to any man.

The most obvious example of my father hunger was Ray.

Everybody Loves Raymond—or not!

The fall of 1987 was an exciting time. After graduating from high school a year earlier, I was finally going off to college. During my first week in school, I rented an apartment, landed a good job, and began juggling all of the responsibilities of adulthood. But inside, I was still a little girl looking for a father figure to make me feel loved, and one of my professors, Ray, fit the mold perfectly.

The first time our eyes met, it was obvious that Ray was taken aback. He visually locked on with a ga-ga look on his face as I walked across the classroom, and he quickly engaged me in conversation in the hallway after class. He soon began visiting my apartment after school and calling often. At thirty-nine years old, he was twenty years older than I. Strike one. He was not only my professor but also the dean of the college I was attending. Strike two. And he was newly married to his *third* wife. Strike three. Yet foolishly, I didn't throw him out of the game. I played around in that relationship for eighteen months, and I lost big-time—my heart, my dignity, and my self-esteem. I finally came to my senses just months before I was to walk down the aisle to become his *fourth* wife. Although he'd studied to become a priest years before, he showed little interest in spiritual matters. I pestered him to attend church with me once we started living together. He visited once, then encouraged me to just go without him. That was how my own mother had lived from Sunday to Sunday, sitting alone in a pew while her husband stayed home, and I didn't want to follow in her footsteps.

My wake-up call came when I asked Ray if he was willing to have more children once we got married. He responded, "I've already had all the kids I want. Besides, I don't know what kind of mother you'd be." *Ouch!* Although it was a valid concern at the time, his comment stung enough to send me walking out the door. Cutting the physical tie was easy. Cutting the soul tie proved to be far more complex.

Haunted by the Ghost of Ray

Fast forward the tape a couple of years. Greg and I had been married only a few months, but reality was already setting in. The marital bliss was wearing thin. Things weren't so hunky-dory anymore. Marriage was proving to be much harder than I thought. And when I wanted to talk to someone about my fears and frustrations, guess whom I naturally gravitated toward? Call me crazy, but yep, I ran back to Ray. (The old proverb is true—a dog returns to its vomit, and a fool returns to his folly![2]) Ray's best response to my disillusionment? "I could have told you that a woman like you would never be happy with a virgin."

Greg's sexual performance hadn't been an issue at all. But Ray's comment stuck with me. One day while Greg and I were about to make love, I pleaded, "I wish you'd approach me with more whirlwind passion! Come on! Sweep me off my feet!"

Greg lovingly but firmly replied, "Shannon, don't ever compare me to someone you had no business being in a sexual relationship with in the first place." Yet another *Ouch!* moment in Shannon Ethridge's colorful history. The truth often hurts, even when it is spoken in love. I had been mentally reminiscing about all of the romantic things Ray had done to make me feel special, yet I was failing to remember just how dysfunctional our "love" for each other had been! I apologized to Greg, and banished memories of Ray from our bedroom.

A few years later, I was having one of those dark days that every stay-at-home mom has on occasion. My kids weren't behaving. The house wasn't staying clean. I had no idea what to make for dinner. And not even Calgon could take me away from the depression that was setting up shop in my spirit as my children stomped on my one last intact nerve. In my mind, I could almost hear Ray's words all over again. "I'm not sure what kind of mother you'd be." It had been years since he'd spoken those words, yet it had obviously stuck in my spirit and traveled through life with me, like a big wad of bubble gum permanently affixed to the bottom of my shoe.

That's when I woke up from that relationship a second time, recognizing that I could no longer be haunted by the ghost of Ray—not in my bedroom, or in my living room, or in any other corner of my mind. He was not an expert in my life, or a wise counselor, or spiritual guru. He was not my father, or even a good example of what a father should be. He was not my soul mate. He was merely a blip on my sexual screen, there to alert me to a painful lesson I needed to learn. I'd carelessly placed my hope and trust in the hands of a man who was only using me to serve his selfish sexual agenda. It was time to cut that thread from my life's tapestry so that it didn't shape any further dysfunctional patterns. Memories of Ray became merely spiritual markers of where I'd once been and how far I'd come since then.

But sometimes life lessons resurface when we fail to firmly remain on the path of inner peace, and the refresher course can be even more painful. A decade after cutting all soul ties with Ray, I walked right into another inappropriate relationship with another married man, who was also twenty years my senior, who was also in authority over me, who had also been like a father figure for many years, who had not only studied to be a minister but was currently serving as one. The most obvious common denominator in my relationships with Ray and with this man, however, was *me*. Obviously, I hadn't completely learned every facet of the lesson my soul was trying to teach me earlier in life, and this was the relationship that sent Greg and me running away to that bed-and-breakfast I mentioned at the opening of this chapter. We needed time away to dissect the dysfunction and figure out an escape plan.

For years, I'd run to John as a spiritual mentor. We frequently had business meetings over lunch as we planned summer camps together. But gradually, more time was spent talking about personal matters than ministry matters. I justified the relationship in my mind, thinking that because it was only an emotional affair, it wasn't as dangerous. Yet it posed the biggest threat to my marriage that I'd ever faced when John suggested, "I'd leave my marriage and ministry if you'd run away to Jamaica with me." For a brief moment, running off with this spiritually wise, adoring man sounded so appealing—like forever sitting beneath the shade of the tree of knowledge. On the other hand, I knew that I'd most likely wind up committing suicide once I realized that I'd done something as stupid as leaving a wonderful husband and two precious children to hang out on a remote island with an insecure little boy trapped in an old man's body. Thankfully, I learned the lesson. He was not my father. He was not my best friend. He was not my spiritual mentor, or my pathway to God. He was not the balm that would soothe my aching soul. He was a stumbling block, and I cleared my path of him by moving one hundred miles away, establishing a "no contact" rule, and cutting all soul ties with him. As a result, my sexual confidence has soared over the past decade.

We all have our own life lessons that our soul longs to teach us, but mine is this: *There is a very fine line between spirituality and sexuality, and my hunger for a father figure is really a hunger to be divinely led by a Higher Power.* In my ignorance of this important lesson, my craving for a deep, soul-to-soul connection with another being is what's led me down many sexually inappropriate roads. But I learned that I don't need a middleman to get in touch with my spirituality, especially not one that's going to lust after my body. I can approach my Higher Power directly and experience spiritual intimacy both on my own and with my husband as we enjoy sex as an act of spiritual worship.

Of course, Ray and John are only a couple of examples of many soul ties I could write about in this chapter. Other women tell me about their soul ties, too, or about the scarlet letter they still wear as a way of punishing themselves for what they've done. For example:

- After her ten-year high school reunion, Charlotte began regularly interacting with an old boyfriend who'd taken her to the prom. Feeling as if her husband was no longer sexually desirous of her, she got her ego stroked from her old boyfriend's reminiscing about how beautiful she looked in her prom dress and how much fun they'd had fooling around in the backseat of his car their senior year. "He says I'm still as sexy as ever," Charlotte gushed, unaware that she's not tiptoeing through the tulips here. She's treading on thin ice.

- Courtney writes, "I was raised with pornography all around, and began acting it out with boys at a very young age. I felt convicted to change, but I didn't know how. Throughout my teen years I remained entrenched in a guilt-inducing lifestyle of indiscriminate sex with a handful of boyfriends. Then I got married as a young adult and slowly began to realize how much my previous relationships left undeniable marks on me—not physically (although one did give me an STD) but more mentally and emotionally. I married a wonderful guy, but I can't have sex with him without thinking that this is the same thing I did with my old boyfriends, and all the guilt from my past just comes flooding into my bedroom, putting a damper on all my sexual desires."

- On an all-girl trip to Vegas, Andrea wound up drinking a little too much, flirting with a fellow poker player all night, and going back to his hotel room. Although her husband knows nothing about this one-night stand, it has been troubling Andrea for months. "I didn't realize that giving that man my body just one time would mean that he dwells in my mind and spirit forever! Oh, how I wish I could live that night over again, do the right thing, and walk out of that casino with my head held high." Every time her husband compliments her or tries to initiate sex, one question plagues Andrea: *Would he still love me if he knew what I've done?* Doubting that he would ever understand and fearing a public scandal that would cause her to lose her job, home, and children, Andrea has resigned herself to carrying this secret to her grave, coping with her lack of sexual confidence as best she can by wearing her happy mask and going through the motions. However, she does occasionally fantasize about a fresh new start with a new husband, thinking she might not have to carry this boatload of guilt in *his* presence.

- Tammy, who had two abortions and multiple partners prior to marriage, once wrote a confession and tucked it into her journal, which was eventually stored in the attic. Her husband of eighteen months came across it, and because this was all shocking news to him, he began doing more research into her past. He hired someone to pull up all of her old e-mails and cell phone calls and found more dirt than he expected. Even though her inappropriate behavior had ceased prior to their dating, her husband feels very threatened by these revelations. He's become verbally and emotionally abusive, and frequently accuses her of fantasizing about old lovers when they are having sex. Unfortunately, Tammy feels she deserves such treatment. She says, "This is just my lot in life. Men will never appreciate me for who I am after all that I've done."

Rather than looking at the life lessons their souls are trying to teach them, these women are doing what so many women do—they are hiding behind a mask rather than getting real with themselves and their husbands, sticking their heads in the sand as to what their actions and feelings could be trying to reveal, sweeping all of their sexual and emotional fears and insecurities under a rug, missing out on genuine marital intimacy and surrendering their sexual self-confidence without a fight.

Have you fallen into this pattern? Perhaps considering these questions can help you discern whether or not this is so:

- Have you resigned yourself to the idea that relational discord and unfulfilled longings are simply your lot in life?
- Do you view yourself through the tainted lens of premarital or extramarital sexual misconduct?

- Do you feel you must keep your sexual activities and feelings a secret so that you will not be judged or rejected?
- Are there men whose phone numbers or e-mail addresses you still have memorized because of your excessive use of them in the past?
- Are there items, photographs, or letters that you hold on to as a reminder of a past premarital or extramarital sexual relationship?
- Do you go out of your way to stroll down the memory lane that you've created with a man other than your husband?

If you answered positively to any of these questions, it may be time for you to get the scarlet letter off your sweater and cut the soul ties that are binding you from becoming a sexually confident wife! How? Just like in the previous chapter, let's take it one step at a time.

"There's a saying in the recovery movement: 'You are only as sick as your secrets.' This is true for relationships as well. If there are secrets that haven't been shared, topics that can't be discussed, things from the past that are forbidden to be brought up, it can cripple a marriage."
—*Rob Bell*, Sex God: Exploring the Endless Connections Between Sexuality and Spirituality

TEN STEPS TOWARD SEXUAL FREEDOM

1. Admit that your sexual identity needs reshaping.

Nothing ever gets fixed as long as we deny that it's broken. Listen to your life. Hear what your soul is trying to say. Let your sexual choices and feelings guide you into a greater level of wisdom and self-understanding. It's okay to feel sexually broken or to have soul ties that still need cutting. However, it's not okay to stay there, ignoring your need for healing and freedom.

2. Make your own list.

As painful as the process may be, a comprehensive list of all romantic pursuits and sexual encounters will reveal a great deal. For each partner, ask yourself, "Why did I have sex with him?" or "Why was I romantically involved with that person at all?" Work your way down the list one person at a time, making note of your responses.

3. Identify the theme.

Once your list is made, take an honest look at the big picture. What common themes become evident? What do most of these men (or women) have in common? What does that tell you?

4. Learn the lesson.

Based on what you've learned so far, what revelations are you able to receive? Do you recognize what it is that you've really been looking for? What area of neediness have you been trying to satisfy through dysfunctional relationships? How has that worked for you?

5. Forgive others.

While it's easy to throw a stone at all of the people on our list for using or abusing us, we have to recognize that in many instances, we've taught them how to treat us. It takes two to tango, and we all play a part in the dance of dysfunction. A healthy woman wouldn't have fallen prey to an unhealthy man's schemes. Ignoring our part and harboring resentment toward him for his part is like *you* drinking poison while hoping *he* dies. Such bitterness does you no good. Do yourself a favor. Forgive the people on your list. Declare that they don't owe you anything. Acknowledge that they were most likely in the same boat as you—seeking to medicate their own emotional pain while clueless as to what damage was really being done.

6. Forgive yourself.

Forgiving everyone else but harboring resentment toward yourself isn't going to fully sever any soul ties. If you truly want to be free, you have to extend forgiveness toward the one your choices have hurt the most—yourself. If you're like me, you were really just a little girl trapped in a grown woman's body when you experienced all those sexual encounters. Forgive that little girl for being so hungry for attention and affection. Give her what her heart's been yearning for all along—unconditional love and acceptance.

7. Create a "no contact" rule.

The worst thing you can do is go down your list and try to contact all of those old partners, even if it's under the guise of "asking forgiveness" from them. That makes about as much sense as an alcoholic returning to all of his favorite bars to say to the bartenders, "I'm sorry I came in here. I'm not going to drink anymore." The bartender is thinking, *Oh, yeah? So why are you here?* If you're really serious about cutting all soul ties, you'll let go of any need you feel to reconnect with previous partners, regardless of how noble your reasons for wanting to do so may seem.

8. Create a "no comparison" rule.

Forgive me if you're offended by my conservative values, but if we weren't married to the people we previously had sex with, we had no business having sex with them. And we certainly have no business dragging a boatload of soul ties and sexual baggage into the bedroom we share with our husbands. Commit to avoiding all comparisons of your husband to past partners—mentally, emotionally, physically, or spiritually. Allow your husband to be the unique individual that he is, not the lesser version of someone else you've known.

9. Keep your slate clean.

Now that you're aware of just how much residue remains after an inappropriate relational encounter, avoid deep emotional connections with any man you aren't married to. Establish firm boundaries in your work and social relationships such that you don't find yourself in the middle of an emotional or sexual affair ever again.

10. Forget intensity and focus on intimacy.

Maybe these suggestions make you feel as if you are going on an emotional starvation diet. *Not reconnect with old boyfriends? Not flirt with my male coworkers? Not meet new men in chat rooms? Can't I have any fun?* Yes, you can, but not at your own heart's expense, which is ultimately what happens when we create inappropriate soul ties. I know that such relational trysts create a lot of intensity, but intensity doesn't last. Intimacy does. Focus on getting to know your spouse even better than you already do, and knowing yourself better. Invest your energies into spicing up your own love life rather than trying to create a new one. And when you are successful, your level of sexual confidence will soar!

Find a Little Help from a Friend

Perhaps you're reading these steps toward sexual freedom and thinking, *There's no way I can be that honest with myself! I don't think I want to know the real truth, because the truth hurts!* Indeed, facing the truth can hurt, but not nearly as much as ignoring it and letting history repeat itself.

If you need a friend to gently take you by the hand and usher you through these steps toward healing, don't hesitate to reach out to one. Try a professional therapist, or a pastoral counselor. If you need a referral, call 1-800-NEW-LIFE. Seek out a female Sex & Love Addicts Anonymous (SLAA) group (www.slaafws.org) or a Celebrate Recovery (CR) group (www.celebraterecovery.com), both of which meet in local churches all over the nation. You don't have to suffer in silence. Connect with a counselor or trusted confidante and cut those soul ties that have bound you for too long. •

Let Your Soul Lead You

I believe hungry souls are like vacuums, supernaturally drawing into our lives people that have lessons we subconsciously need to learn. However, once we learn the lesson, we can release the individuals completely. We don't owe them anything, and neither do they owe us anything. We can look at the relationship as a spiritual marker of where we once were in life. We can forgive one another for the pain we've caused, then move on with incredibly valuable lessons tucked safely in the pocket of our hearts—lessons that will serve us well as we continue striving to be the best wives we can be.

We simply do not have to be bound by soul ties to people that no longer enhance our lives. We aren't required to keep in contact with those who prevent us from being our best selves. We can let go. We can move on. We can experience true sexual freedom. We can be emotionally faithful, sexually confident wives who bring joy and comfort into the lives of everyone around us. And we can share our life's lessons with those who are still on their journey toward wisdom and inner peace, helping all of our sisters understand what fantastic females we really are.

Part 3

The Fantastic Sexual Female

6

Harnessing Your Sexual Power

After twelve years of living in the concrete jungle of Dallas, Texas, I was ready for a change. A log cabin home on 122 acres of land was just the cure for our traffic-weary souls. As I envisioned what country life would be like, I became obsessed with one thing—*riding horses!* I frequently pictured myself atop a dappled gray mare, galloping through wildflower-laden fields bursting with color, the wind whipping through my hair, like a scene out of a movie.

Once we were settled in our country home, we noticed that our neighbor's pasture was lit up like a professional ballpark every Thursday night. Curious, we ventured over to introduce ourselves one evening, and I almost did a backflip when I realized that the lights were illuminating their own rodeo arena! Bob and Lisa owned a slew of horses, training calf ropers and barrel racers as a hobby, as well as breeding horses professionally for a living. Imagine my delight the day that Bob asked, "Would you mind taking care of my horses for a few days while we're in New Mexico? You can throw a saddle on one and take her for a ride whenever you want." Gee, Bob. Twist my arm.

Bob and Lisa hadn't been gone half an hour before I called my friend and ecstatically exclaimed, "Come over and ride horses with us!" Katie brought her three kids, and the seven of us took turns all afternoon riding Yeller, the only horse we managed to catch.

With the sun creeping further west, we knew it was time to hang up our reins and call it a day. Katie offered me the last ride, and I enthusiastically mounted Yeller with the expectation that all my equestrian dreams were about to come to fruition. We started off at a turtle pace, but with a double click of my tongue in the roof of my mouth, I coaxed Yeller into a slightly higher gear. We trotted for a few moments, but I wanted more. I wanted wind in my face. So I let out my best "Heeyaa!" and buried the heel of my boots in Yeller's belly. Suddenly, we were off and running at breakneck speed, my hair flapping in rhythm with every thunderous gallop. I was basking in the exhilaration of it all, but then my basking turned to bewilderment as the horizon suddenly tilted sideways and the sky went black.

After several seconds of unconsciousness, I awoke to the realization that my saddle had slid sideways, dumping me face-first onto the dirt and dragging me for several yards before the stirrup loosened its death grip on my foot. I remember my desperation the moment I realized that the reins were no longer in my hands. Without a firm grip on that harness, there was absolutely no way to control that horse. I thought I was taking Yeller for the ride of my life, but she almost took me for the *last* ride of my life.

Our sex drive holds a similar power. On the one hand, it can add great passion and pleasure to our lives, satisfying our deepest needs for intimate connection and fulfilling our wildest dreams. On the other hand, it also holds the power to create enormous pain and fear, turning our lives into a living nightmare if we fail to keep a tight hold on the reins.

Losing Control of the Sexual Reins

Although we've historically considered sexual infidelity a "man's issue," women are actually falling into extramarital affairs at almost the same astounding rate (40–65 percent, depending on which study you're looking at). With many women working alongside men outside the home, traveling frequently, carrying cell phones and Black-Berries, and so on, it's more convenient than ever to have a boy toy on the side.

While one might imagine that a woman who pursues or gets involved in an extramarital affair is a "sexually confident" woman, I beg to differ. I've attempted to drink from that stream, and it wasn't because I was sexually confident. It was because I lacked confidence and had to look elsewhere for the affirmation that I couldn't find within myself and my own marriage. Besides, simply being a sexually confident *woman* isn't the goal. The goal is to be a sexually confident *wife*. Our aim is to create a mad, passionate romance and fulfilling love relationship with the man we currently live with and have committed to grow old with. Making love is easy. Making love last is far more challenging.

In fact, some wives (even good wives) experience overwhelming temptation to simply go back to making love with a new man. Sometimes it seems so much easier than trying to make love last with the man she already has.

- Christy e-mails, "In our earliest years of marriage, I was very secure in our relationship, and we were both very happy. But now I find myself searching for approval outside my marriage, and I'm afraid my jealousy and insecurities are going to get the best of me. My husband is a pilot and is extremely friendly with everyone he meets. He is gone from home four to five days per week, and spends evenings going out to eat with other pilots and flight attendants. I sit at home struggling with feelings of not being good enough, so I interact with anyone who'll give me some attention—our painter, the other husbands in the neighborhood, any stranger in cyberspace. I have been dieting and exercising more than I know I should (I am 5'4", 115 lbs.). It is becoming an obsession, and I feel as if lots of men find me attractive, with the exception of my husband. How can I keep from acting out on these overwhelming temptations to engage in an affair?"

Maybe if Christy heard what Janet had to say, she'd rethink the whole affair idea . . .

- Janet writes, "My husband and I were high school sweethearts, and I always assumed there'd never be another man for me. But after a while I began to wonder what I'd missed out on by marrying the first man who asked. I guess you could say my first extramarital affair was a 'seven-year-itch' kind of thing, but it never fully scratched my itch. It opened the door for even more inappropriate relationships, since I felt like I'd already blown the whole fidelity thing. Over the past twelve years, I've had eight affairs, some sexual, some strictly emotional. I wish I could say I've always been the victim of seduction, but I've actually been the seductress in most cases. I live every day of my life worrying that if my husband found out what I'm really like, he'd leave me and take the kids and everything else with him. If he did, I can't say that I'd blame him. I loathe myself on a daily basis, which creates even more temptation to look to another man to make me feel better. I've created a vicious cycle that I don't know how to get out of short of suicide."

Unfortunately, I'm painfully familiar with the kind of desperation these women express. When we use our external beauty and seductive powers to lure men into meeting our emotional needs for attention and affirmation, we assume our insecurities will just sweetly melt away like cotton candy on a child's tongue. But we often create a tumultuous double life when we look to another man to medicate our emotional pain. Once the high of an affair wears off, we frequently find ourselves addicted, going back to our old "junkie" or finding a new one to provide more of our drug of choice. This extramarital high makes it more and more difficult to find satisfaction on the home front.

"I consider promiscuity immoral. Not because sex is evil, but because sex is too good and important."
—Ayn Rand, Russian-American writer

Putting Sexual Power into Perspective

What we're really longing for—genuine passion, intimacy, and connection—can best be found not by looking for a new man but by creating the relationship of our dreams with the man we already have. Rather than relentlessly searching for the ideal lover, let's simply create the ideal love.

How is that possible? Here are five guidelines to help you harness your sexual power and use it for the greater good of your marriage relationship.

1. Recognize the enormous power your sexuality holds.

The one aspect that sets your marriage relationship apart from all others is sexual intimacy. No matter how close we are with our parents, children, or best friends, we can only go so deep in those relationships. In marriage, however, intimacy knows no boundaries. The more intimately our bodies are touched, the more deeply our hearts and souls are touched. The more our bodies are neglected or abused by each other, the more deeply our hearts and souls are scarred.

Some women say they want the marriage without the sex, or vice versa. However, a marriage without sex is nothing more than a live-in friendship. And a sexual relationship without a marriage commitment is just a temporary thrill and a heartache waiting to happen. But a husband and wife giving freely of themselves to arouse and satisfy each other in a way that no one else on the planet is allowed to is an incredibly powerful thing. It's like sexual cement that forms the pillars of a strong family and society. Be a good steward of that sexual relationship, placing it on a plane above all others.

2. Never withhold sex as punishment for bad behavior.

Occasionally I'll see a report on the news about parents who severely neglect or abuse "bad" children by withholding a basic need such as nutritious food or medicine when they are ill. Perhaps you've heard of such examples as well, and if you're like me, it's enraged you. We wonder, *How could someone abuse their power by withholding a genuine need from someone they love?*

In all honesty, I've wondered the same thing at times when we receive e-mails from husbands bewildered by their wives' withholding of sex. Of course, there are times when a woman is being abused herself and is withholding sex as a self-protective mechanism, but I'm not talking about that. I'm referring to situations when women are simply overlooking what a basic need sex is for their husbands and choosing to abuse their power by withholding their bodies as punishment for some petty behavior they don't appreciate. While you may feel justified in doing this at times, thinking it's not that big of a deal to him, keep in mind that some husbands would sooner give up food or shelter before they'd choose to give up sex. If you love him, show him by sharing your body freely with him—no strings attached.

3. View sex as much more than just a reward for good behavior.
A woman is naturally more prone to initiate physical affection when she is pleased with her husband's performance. When he goes above and beyond to help you in the house or make you feel special, or gets a promotion at work, or really goes the extra mile in spending quality time with the kids, it's easy to want to toss him a cookie.

However, women have to be careful not to reduce sex to a doggie treat that's handed out only when he does the right tricks or obeys our commands. He'll catch on to that quickly, and while he loves the treats, he'll come to resent the hoops he's expected to jump through to get them. The sexually confident wife doesn't keep her husband on a short sexual leash with the expectation that he'll heed her every instruction. She initiates sex with him simply because she loves him and wants him to know it, even when his performance isn't necessarily worthy of special attention. Besides, awarding sex only when he pays the right price causes a wife to more closely resemble a prostitute than a life partner. Remember, your sexual relationship isn't about what you accomplish for each other. It's about who you are and what you mean to each other.

4. Avoid the old "bait and switch" trick.

"I don't understand why my wife finds _____ such a repulsive act when she seemed more than happy to do that when we were dating. I feel like she pulled the old 'bait and switch' trick on me!" Sadly, my husband and I have heard this sentiment expressed on numerous occasions. Women often wield their sexual power by doing anything their boyfriend desires to get them hooked. But after the wedding band goes on her finger, she rewrites the sexual rulebook. By making certain acts against the rules, she is basically saying to her husband, "That's gross. And you're gross for wanting to do that. I must have married a pervert." And what does this do to his sexual confidence? Let's just say that if his feelings were visible and audible, we'd see him wince and hear him yell, *"Ouch!"*

One of the worst uses of our sexual power is to use it to insult or inflict harm on our husbands. If there are sexual activities you've engaged in together previously that you no longer feel comfortable with, verbalize why you feel the way you do and make sure he does not feel judged for enjoying that act. Talk it through with the goal of reaching a compromise that you can both feel good about. Chapter 11 will help you establish a set of sexual boundaries that feel comfortable for you, and will help you respectfully communicate those as well.

5. Don't keep score in the bedroom.

"Sex is always all about you! It's never about me and what I want!" While many women may have the right to feel that way, harshly verbalizing such a sentiment isn't the greatest of aphrodisiacs. A friend once informed her husband that they'd only be having sex when they had the time and energy for them both to reach orgasm. What did this do to their sex life? Quite frankly, it killed it. While they used to have sex at least once each week, it became more like once every six weeks or so, then she admitted to me that it had been six months! When I asked what she was getting out of this little game, she replied, "I'm keeping the score even."

Consider two women—one who gives far more than she receives sexually (but doesn't keep score) and the other who plays this "tit for tat" game (no pun intended). Which one of them is really the winner in her marriage? The one who demands every bit as much attention as she gives, or the one who gives freely? The sexually insecure wife keeps score and demands equality. But the sexually confident wife knows that it's more blessed to give than to receive, for that is how we inspire (rather than require) intimacy in a relationship.

The Prize of Harnessed Power

When a wife feels confident that she can avoid extramarital affairs, when she recognizes the incredible power her sexuality holds to create a supernatural bond in her marriage, when she refrains from manipulative games such as withholding sex for bad behavior, using sex to reward good behavior, playing the "bait and switch" trick, or keeping score in the bedroom, then she's harnessing her sexual power. What's the prize? The ability to create that wonderfully intimate relationship she's dreamed of.

This chapter was introduced with a horse analogy, and I want to close it with yet another image: that of a flowing river. If a river overflows its banks, it has immense destructive power. Homes can be flooded, families separated, and even lives lost. But by remaining within its banks, that flowing river brings life and blessings to every village or community it serves.

Inappropriate use of sexual power can have a similar effect, emotionally and spiritually destroying homes, families, and lives. But by harnessing your sexual power and keeping it within the appropriate boundaries, you can also bring a renewed sense of life and blessings to your marriage and family. Rather than requiring a fulfilling relationship with your husband, you'll naturally inspire it. And when that happens, your heart and body may gravitate closer to your husband than ever before, giving you both a new, powerful sense of sexual confidence.

7

Befriending the Body Image Bear

"Can you lead me to the Sexuality section of your store?"

The question obviously elicited fear and trepidation in the middle-aged female salesclerk. With a deer-in-the-headlights look on her face, she ushered me three rows over from the customer service desk, then halfway down the aisle. She pointed to dozens, if not hundreds of books on the topic of sex. She laughed and said, "These are the most stolen titles in our collection. We find the book jackets in the bathroom trash cans frequently."

Curious as to what else had been written on the topic of sexual confidence, I was overwhelmed by so many titles to peruse. I asked the woman which books she recommended. She responded emphatically, "Oh, I wouldn't know! I don't read these books! I'm divorced now, but if my husband had brought one of these home for me to read, I would have just looked at him like he'd lost his mind!"

My curiosity was piqued, so I decided to fish a little. "Do you mind my asking why you feel that way?"

"Have you seen the women in these books? That's just not me! I don't look anything like those women," she replied. "I'd rather wrestle a bear than look at one of those books."

I couldn't imagine where this woman was coming from. Standing at about 5'5", her petite frame couldn't have weighed more than 120 pounds soaking wet. Size six would be my best guess, a size most women would kill to get into. Somewhat confused, I thanked her for her time, then searched the stacks and selected about twenty titles to glance through.

As I sat in my comfy chair in the middle of the store, I slowly began to understand this woman's sentiment. Page after page, book after book, there "she" was. *The perfect woman.* Long hair flowing down around her perky, round, symmetrical breasts, flat tummy untainted by stretch marks or post-pregnancy pounds, slender hips and firm derriere, shapely thighs without a hint of cellulite. Not one unsightly scar, pimple, or spider vein on her whole body. Just one hundred or so pounds of graceful, seductive energy.

Before I made it through the first three books, I found myself preferring to wrestle a bear as well. But then I realized I *was* wrestling a bear—*the body image bear*—the mental image that sends so many women running for a safe hiding place (usually behind baggy sweats or fuzzy robes), surrendering their sexual confidence every step of the way. That's when I realized how my book needed to be different from all the others. Only by including sketches of *real women*—ripples, rolls, wrinkles, and all (which you'll find in Chapter 10), could I convince every female that she deserves to be a sexually confident wife.

Never Good Enough

The interesting thing about body image is that no matter how good we might look, we always think we should look better. Perhaps that's because 75 percent of female sitcom characters we look at from week to week on television are underweight, not to mention the airbrushed anorexic cover models we have to stare at every time we go to buy a jug of milk (skim or 1 percent of course). It's a rather unfair comparison when you consider that the average American woman is 5'4" and weighs 140 pounds, yet the average American model is 5'11" and weighs 117 pounds.[1]

But many of those models and celebrities, some of the sexiest, most enviable women of our day, often feel as if they have a long way to go before they are good enough. Although she's been voted the sexiest, most beautiful woman alive by many publications, Scarlett Johansson was quoted as saying, "Everyone in Hollywood is so damn skinny. You constantly feel like you're not skinny enough."[2] Print and runway model Kate Dillon had to take time off from her career to work on her body because she was told she was too large to be a model (even though she was already underweight). *Ally McBeal's* Calista Flockhart finally admitted after years of denial that she had an eating disorder, abusing her body by overexercising and undereating.[3] When women like Scarlett Johansson, Kate Dillon, and Calista Flockhart aren't good enough in their own eyes, it's easy to wonder how the heck we are supposed to feel about our own fuller-figured selves. In fact, most women aren't satisfied with themselves at all. According to the National Eating Disorders Association,

- approximately 45 percent of women are dieting on any given day (the rest are probably just taking a day off).
- 80 percent of women report that they are unhappy with their appearance (and when Mama ain't happy, ain't nobody happy).[4]

And how does this dissatisfaction with our weight and low self-esteem affect our sexual confidence? *USA Today* reports that the number one reason women avoid sex is—(drumroll, please)—because they feel uncomfortable with how their body looks.[5] *No! Really?* Okay, maybe you're not so shocked by that news flash. Neither was I. Most of us have been there, done that, got the T-shirt and the video. And the T-shirt was too small, which fueled our belief that we are simply too fat.

So why are women so hard on themselves, even those who are relatively healthy and look fantastic by most standards? Perhaps it's because we've bought the lie that men want pencil-thin, couldn't-pinch-an-inch-if-their-life-depended-on-it kind of women. But I want to let you in on a little secret: *Although women may not like their curves, men love them!*

Don't believe me? Listen to what a few of our male friends said to my husband and me as I was writing this book . . .

"Women who have no meat on their bones don't look like women at all. They look like prepubescent girls. Those stick figures may appeal to the perverts out there, but I want a full-grown woman, with a full-grown body. I want someone whose round curves I can drink in through my eyes and trace over with my fingertips."
—Herb, age 44

"My wife may weigh a bit more than the typical supermodel, but I wouldn't have it any other way. I love how she looks. So as long as she's happy with herself, I'm great."
—Paul, age 37

"I don't want to buy a girl a twenty-dollar meal only to have her pick at it and eat one-tenth of it because she doesn't want to get fat. Give me a break. She probably goes home and eats half a cheesecake

because she's starving by the end of the evening. Give me a woman
with some hips, some thighs, and an appetite for good food and fun."
—Dave, age 25

"My wife's hips have gotten a little wider through the years, and her
breasts may have fallen a little southward since I fell in love with her
more than thirty years ago. But when I consider the four beautiful
children who've passed through those hips and nursed at those
breasts, I'm more in awe of them than ever. To everyone else, she's a
grandma. To me, she's a goddess, and I celebrate her
presence in my life every day."
—Terry, age 59

Men frequently seem desperate to help their wives understand that
their bodies are beautiful just the way they are. Of course, you don't
have to struggle with excess weight to wrestle the image bear. Sometimes he attacks from the opposite end of the spectrum. Kathy writes:

> I've struggled with an eating disorder for about twenty years.
> I'm not severely underweight or bulimic, but I long to be free
> from the constant preoccupation with my body. I know it robs
> me of my sexual confidence, as I can never just accept the fact
> that my husband thinks I'm attractive (mainly because I don't
> think I'm attractive). But like the chicken and the egg thing,
> I have to wonder, *Which came first?* My eating disorder or my
> sexual insecurities?

Regardless of which came first, I believe both of these body image
bears can be slain with the help of a good counselor, so don't hesitate
to seek one out if you can sympathize with Kathy's struggles.

Perhaps weight issues aren't what hinders your sexual confidence at all, but rather a certain part of your body. Retta shares:

> When it comes to breasts, I wish I were more blessed. I try on sexy lingerie and the breast pocket just hangs there, as I don't have enough to even fill an A cup completely. I've thought about breast implants but am not comfortable with the risks involved. My husband says he loves my small breasts, but you never see women in pornographic movies with small breasts, so I can't help but wonder if he's lying just to make me feel better.

Regardless of what you see most often in magazines and movies, there are plenty of men who love small breasts, and if your husband is one of them, don't question his judgment. Learn to take his compliments at face value rather than searching for some lie lurking behind his sentiments. Which reminds me of a message I was asked to deliver one time . . .

A Message to All Wives

In the spring of 2007, I spoke in Edmonton, Alberta, Canada, at an intergenerational sexuality conference where women gathered at one location and men gathered at a nearby venue. On Saturday afternoon, the male speaker and I switched places, allowing me the opportunity to address the men for one session. As I was leaving the building to return to the women's conference, one tall man with a weathered complexion and a worried look on his face asked if he could have one moment of my time.

"When you go back to speak to the ladies, will you deliver a message to all of them, my wife especially?" he asked.

"Sure. What's on your heart?" I asked.

He replied, "Please tell them that they *don't* have to be modest." Suddenly his eyes filled with tears, and he explained, "I've been trying to tell my wife for eighteen years that she's beautiful, but she won't believe me. She makes me feel like I must be crazy to think she's sexy, and sometimes I'm tempted to just believe her. But I refuse to do that. I want her to believe me instead. I know what I see when I look at her. I just want her to feel the same way about herself."

I fought back my own tears as I sensed this man's gnawing pain and growing frustration. As I delivered that message to the women in the next session, I sensed that every female in the crowd wondered if it was from her own husband. Every woman seemed to acknowledge her own guilt in this matter. We've all questioned our own sexual attractiveness, and questioned our husband's sanity if he disagreed with our negative assessment. This breaks my heart.

"There is but one temple in the Universe . . . and that is the human body. Nothing is holier than that high form. We touch heaven when we lay our hand on the human body."
—*Thomas Carlyle, British historian*

We must remember that beauty is in the eye of the beholder, and in a marriage relationship, there are two sets of eyes beholding your naked body—your husband's and your own. Joy comes from knowing that the two of you are seeing the exact same thing—a beautiful, sexually confident woman, a woman whose inner attitudes about herself carry far more weight than any external factor.

On *Saturday Night Live,* Billy Crystal (mimicking Fernando Lamas) frequently used to say, "It's not important how you feel, dahling. It's how you look, and you look ma-a-a-hvelous!" But the reverse is far more accurate. What you look like isn't nearly as important as how you feel about yourself. It's not your perfectly proportioned assets but your perfectly confident attitude that floats his boat the most.

Granted, if your weight has gotten out of control and you've truly let yourself go, you are going to feel much better about yourself after you start to look better. But when you've done all you can do toward that end (excluding starving yourself or undergoing plastic surgery), you owe it to yourself to be pleased with your personal best, which is going to look different from someone else's personal best because we are all unique. But I believe every woman should be able to look into the mirror, appreciate the beauty of what she sees, and be proud to share that precious gift freely with her husband—stretch marks, C-section scars, cellulite, and all. Let's take a lesson from Lacey, who e-mailed:

> We've been married five years, and my daughter is three. I gained a lot of weight when I was pregnant, which affected my self-esteem. However, when I'm having sex with my husband, I feel totally uninhibited, and for that little bit of time, I forget how I look or how much I dislike my excess pounds. When my husband tells me I am beautiful and that he loves me and desires me, I may not always understand why, but I never doubt it. I can be sexually confident because I am confident in his feelings for me. I know my husband enjoys sex with me no matter what I look like. I think you can be a little dissatisfied with your body but still be a very sexually confident wife.

Indeed, you can be a sexually confident wife regardless of your size or shape! If you long to feel more confident, here are my top ten tactics for defeating the body image bear the next time he challenges you to a mental wrestling match.

TOP 10 POSITIVE BODY IMAGE TACTICS

1. Rid your mind of sexual stereotypes.

Because of the media images we are bombarded with, it's easy to believe that sexual confidence is only for the young, thin glamour girl. *Bzzzt!* Sorry, not so. I've known some very large women who are extremely sexually confident, as well as some tiny waifs who cower at the thought of undressing in front of anyone. Also, older women often describe themselves as more sexually confident than younger ones, so age is irrelevant as well. All humans can be sexually confident with the right attitude, so celebrate your sexuality regardless of the numbers on your bathroom scale, tape measure, or birth certificate.

My mental stereotype of "sexy" was shattered when I was working on a master's degree in counseling and human relations. In the textbook for my human sexuality class, I discovered the most beautifully erotic picture I've ever laid eyes on. This wasn't the typical Abercrombie & Fitch–type photo of a young studmuffin with six-pack abs and a beautiful blonde who went through puberty two hours earlier. Rather, an elderly couple, most likely in their seventies or eighties, were fully disrobed (naked!) and freely engaging in passionate foreplay. While a teenager may have barfed to imagine that Grandma and Grandpa might still do such a thing, I was encouraged. I thought, *Wow! She's gorgeous! And like her, I never have to "outgrow" my sexual confidence, regardless of how old, flabby, or wrinkled I become.* And I was right. I don't intend to outgrow my sexuality—ever. And I hope you don't either.

> "I feel that the older I get, the more shameless I feel.
> And in a sense, more pure."
> —Maria Irene Fornes, American playwright

2. Don't assume that your husband is pointing out your flaws every time he touches you.

Sometimes we are so self-conscious about our body that we assume everyone else is focusing on the negatives as well, especially Hubby. But before you make him sleep on the couch because he pinched one of your inches, consider this . . . He may be caressing your love handles, squeezing your thighs, or patting your bottom simply because he thinks they are cute, so take it as a compliment. It's far better that he wants to touch you than not.

Most men don't expect perfection from their wives because they don't have the perfect body, either. Yes, our male counterparts have their own body image hang-ups—undefined abs, beer bellies, love handles, too much back and butt hair, not enough head and chest hair; they fear they are too short and too pale, and that their penis length and circumference aren't sufficient. The only difference between men and women is that men don't usually let these insecurities dampen their sexual confidence. Let's learn from them, ladies.

3. Take a healthy inventory.

Sure, there are plenty of body parts that seem problematic at first glance in the mirror. For most women, it's the parts that naturally change during our baby-making years—hips, tummy, breasts, and so on. But chances are, you've got far more parts that you are pleased or at least satisfied with than not. Undress and stand up straight and tall in front of a full-length mirror. Start from the top of your head and go all the way to the tips of your toes. How do you feel about your hair, eyes, nose, smile, ears, jawline? Your shoulders, arms, elbows, wrists, hands, fingers, fingernails? Your chest, ribs, belly button, spine? Thighs, knees, calves, ankles, feet, toes, toenails?

Rather than focus on the few negatives all of the time, find the positives and introduce your internal commentator (that voice inside your head that never shuts up) to them. Insist that she compliment you about the good parts far more often than she criticizes your other parts. For example, I used to beat myself up over the "spare tire" that seemed to encircle my midsection—from my lower abdomen, around my hips, and my derriere. But one day I noticed that my breasts were full and round—the kind that many women pay big bucks to have artificially installed—and I smiled. Lately I've noticed how my outer thighs and calves are extremely well defined for a woman my age (heck, for a woman of any age), and I decided that I really like my legs. Someone said to me recently, "You could be a foot model!" Rather than say, "No! Look at this scar on my toe!" I simply replied, "Thank you." Now when I look at my feet, I realize that person was right. They are beautiful. Lots of my body parts are beautiful, and I'm allowed to love them. Lots of your parts are beautiful. Learn to love them as well.

"The most common error made in matters of appearance is the belief that one should disdain the superficial and let the true beauty of one's soul shine through. If there are places on your body where this is a possibility, you are not attractive—you are leaking."

—*Fran Lebowitz, writer, humorist*

4. Focus on function, and be grateful.

One of the best things we can do to enhance sexual confidence is to work out regularly. The goal isn't to try to look like a supermodel. Only laxatives create that look, and I can't recommend them. The goal of exercising regularly is to release the wonderful endorphins that are natural mood enhancers and confidence builders.

I know, I know. Working out is hard. But the more you do it, the easier it gets. It even becomes fun if you find activities you enjoy. I used to passionately hate working out. The huge mirrors in the gym seemed more like carnival funhouse mirrors. I'd see my reflection and think, *Surely that's not what I really look like!* As I climbed the Stairmaster, my focus was on my little love handles and post-pregnancy pooch. As I walked on the treadmill, my focus was on my jiggly arms or my bouncing breasts. I left the gym more discouraged than encouraged, even after a great endorphin-producing workout.

However, the older I get, the more I enjoy working out, even though my body is pretty much the same shape and size as it has always been. What's the difference? I focus on function rather than aesthetics. As I walk, climb, row, lift, or stretch, I pay attention to the fluid motion of my body and the strength of the muscles being used. I celebrate the fact that I'm in my forties and all of my body parts work beautifully. That makes me feel attractive, which translates into added sexual confidence.

5. Avoid unrealistic comparisons.

Comparing ourselves to other people is natural but not always healthy. Pay attention to what it does to your self-esteem. For example, if you go to the mall on a Friday night and compare yourself to the teen girls in their low-rise jeans and tight tees, you may find yourself in the dumps before dinnertime. But return the next morning and compare yourself to the blue-haired, arthritic retirees walking laps around the mall in their Reeboks, and your self-esteem will most likely soar.

I'm not throwing a stone here. When I spend all day around my sixteen-year-old daughter's friends, I can get self-conscious about my size and shape if I'm not very careful to guard my thoughts. I have to remember that I'm not sixteen anymore, and I wouldn't go back there again even if you paid me an insane amount of money! But when I used to spend the day visiting my grandparents at the nursing home where they resided, I often returned home feeling like the hottest thing on the planet.

I'm not saying that you *should* compare yourself to other women; I'm just saying that if you do, be fair about it. Don't just compare yourself to younger, thinner girls and allow your sexual confidence to bottom out. Compare yourself to all women on the planet, including the elderly, the morbidly obese, or those who can't function sexually at all due to physical or mental health challenges. Then feel great about all you have to offer your husband (and yourself) sexually.

6. Choose your vocabulary wisely.

Never underestimate the power of your words. They can make everyone around you (especially yourself) feel terrific or terrible. How you talk about yourself teaches other people how to look at you, as well as how to treat you. And the words you use to describe your body can make or break your own sexual confidence.

Therefore, if you have a larger than average physique, don't call yourself "fat" or "chubby." Try "voluptuous" instead. If you're not a frou-frou glamour girl, don't call yourself "plain Jane." You're a "natural beauty." If your breasts are on the small side, don't use the term "flat-chested." Instead, try describing your build as "trim" or "athletic." If your body isn't as toned as you'd like it to be, you don't have to call yourself "flabby." You're just "soft." Lots of men like soft, or trim, or natural, or voluptuous. And they are far more likely to love those attributes when you celebrate them as well.

7. Choose your wardrobe wisely.

Often our lack of sexual confidence stems not from our body but from the clothes we put on it. If you wear something that looks like it was manufactured at Acme Tent & Awning, you're going to feel like the fat lady from the circus. If you put on something that accentuates your curves, you're going to feel far more confident. It doesn't have to be skintight or uncomfortable, just flattering to your shape. Donate any clothes that make you feel fat or frumpy to Goodwill so that the only clothes in your wardrobe will be those that make you feel confident.

Even better than sexy clothing, however, is your beautiful bare skin. Nothing will scream "I'm a sexually confident woman!" like walking around naked whenever you get a chance.

8. Learn to like what you see when you look in the mirror.

Stop approaching the mirror in search of flaws that need fixing. Instead, approach the mirror and take a moment or two to affirm the things you like. Surely you have a few features from the earlier inventory—your hair, your eyes, your nose, your smile, your shoulders, your hourglass shape—that you enjoy looking at. Start with those, and then you can look to see if there is lipstick on your teeth, mascara shadows under your eyes, or a hair out of place. Once you correct that issue, admire the overall package once again and walk away encouraged.

When a woman likes what she sees in the mirror, she exudes an aura that invites others to celebrate what they see when they look in her direction as well. People are often uncomfortable being around a woman who is insecure about her beauty. She feels like a leech, sucking the life out of others as she fishes for the compliment that just might convince her that she does have something—*anything*—worth admiring. Don't be one of those women. Exude confidence.

9. **Learn to love who you see in the mirror.**

Maybe you think I'm being redundant here, but there's a huge difference between *liking what* you see, and *loving who* you see. In my earliest seasons of womanhood, I liked *what* I saw when I looked at my body in the mirror, but I didn't love *who* I saw at all. I had such little love for her that I shared my body too freely, hoping to gain from someone else what I couldn't give myself—true love. It never worked.

In later seasons, I learned to love who I saw (the inside), but I didn't like what I saw (the outside). Age was beginning to take its toll on my body, and in my midthirties I had to come to grips with the fact that I was never going to have the body of a fifteen-year-old again, no matter how hard I exercised or dieted. It seemed all would be downhill from here. But finally, in my early forties, I've learned to do both—love who I am *and* like what I see. Together, there is synergy, and this synergy creates great confidence.

10. **Teach other women how to treat themselves.**

Don't fall into the poor-self-image pit that someone else digs. We often attempt to make others feel better by dragging ourselves to an even lower level. "You think you're fat? Come on! Look at me!" we reply. In the movie *Real Women Have Curves,* four female coworkers begin lamenting about their bodies to one another. The first woman, average in size, says, "Look at me! I'm a cow!"

A slightly larger coworker replies, "If you're a cow, then I'm a hippo!"

The third woman, quite a full-figured gal, retorts, "Well, if you're a hippo, then I'm an elephant!"

The last woman, the most voluptuous one of the bunch, chimes in, "If you're a cow, and you're a hippo, and you're an elephant, then I'm an orca!"

Rather than riding that downward escalator with someone who is bashing her body, reply to her woes with a word of encouragement such as "Hey! Don't talk about my friend that way! I think she's stunningly beautiful just the way she is!" Avoid falling into the pit yourself, and try pulling her out as well.

Don't Worry. Be Happy.

Remember, the perfect body doesn't automatically equate to happiness, and neither do we have to postpone happiness until we have the perfect body. Many celebrities and supermodels have what Hollywood considers the perfect body, but many of those women are never happy with themselves, which means they never feel truly sexually confident. They never win the wrestling match with the body image bear.

Happiness is a choice and you can choose it now. Choosing happiness and self-acceptance can do as much (if not more) for your sexual confidence as losing those ten vanity pounds or getting any surgical procedure done.

Genuine, lasting happiness comes from befriending the body image bear—learning to be content with what we have, who we are, and what we are able to offer those we love. And when a woman can offer her body with confidence that it's something special, regardless of its size or shape, she is offering her husband the most beautiful thing imaginable—a sexually confident wife.

8

Experiencing the Big "Oh!"

here must be something wrong with me. That was the only conclusion my eleven-year-old mind could draw from my mother's response when I asked her, pointing to the inner labia of my vagina, "Why have these flaps of skin gotten bigger?"

"Have you been putting anything inside there?" she asked, looking puzzled.

"No, ma'am."

"Have you been tugging on them?" she inquired further.

"No," I replied honestly.

Her final thoughts on the matter? "Well, I don't know what to tell you. I don't know why they are like that."

I was hoping she could simply tell me, "You're normal," but that wasn't the message I received. Although I know it wasn't her intention, if she had been trying to rob me of my sexual confidence early in life, she would have succeeded. Not that this fear of genital abnormality kept me from becoming sexually active within a few short years, but it certainly kept me from being sexually confident. Most encounters were in a dark room, covers up, him on top, for fear that my freakish monster labia would be discovered. Once I even asked my gynecologist if he'd trim them down surgically. He refused without explanation.

There are several big "Oh!" moments in a woman's life when it comes to understanding and accepting our own bodies. Unfortunately, the one regarding my labia didn't come for almost two decades after fear and trepidation initially set in. In my midthirties, I was taking a master's level human sexuality class, and our textbook contained graphic illustrations of every human body part imaginable. One particular page jumped out at me. Three different pictures of women's vaginal areas adorned the margins. One woman's inner labia were neatly tucked inside her outer labia, similar to what you expect to see when you change a little girl's diaper. This is what I always perceived as "normal," although mine didn't look anything like that. The middle woman's inner labia were a little more pouty, slightly protruded from her outer labia, much like mine. The final picture remedied all my insecurities about being a freak of nature. She looked like something out of a 3-D movie, with her inner labia dangling well outside her vaginal area. Yet all three of these anatomical examples were considered "normal" by health experts.

It sounds crazy, but I proudly displayed the page to my husband, who looked at me as if to say, "And you are showing me this *why?*"

"I'm normal!" I said, beaming.

"Actually, you're pretty abnormal, showing your husband pictures of other women's vaginas!" he replied.

I told him the story of how I felt about my body as I was going through puberty, and confessed that I had carried that mental scar for more than twenty years.

"I've never known that you felt that way," Greg said sweetly.

I probably had more confidence with him than anyone else because I knew mine was the only real vagina he'd ever laid eyes on. (Surely he knew that the porn stars' genitals he had gazed upon as a curious teenager had been airbrushed for effect.) But oh, the euphoric feeling that I experienced when I realized that I truly am normal! Finally, when I heard Greg say, "You're so beautiful," while gazing between my legs, I could actually believe him.

While it may sound silly to carry around a twenty-year fear that you have distorted labia, my guess is that there's probably a body part that you've questioned the normalcy or beauty of. If not your vagina, perhaps it's your other female assets like your breasts, hips, or buttocks that cause insecurities like many of the women we discussed in Chapter 3. My advice is that if your doctor says a body part is normal, take his or her word for it. A doctor won't compare you to a silver screen celebrity or magazine model. A doctor will compare you to all the other real people seen in the examining room.

While all women differ in the sizes and shapes of our body parts and sexual organs, we're not so different when it comes to how those body parts function and what we find pleasurable. Therefore, let's take a look at a few other "Oh!" moments in many women's lives.

The Arousal "Oh!"

Remember when you were a hormonal teenage girl and you'd think to yourself before a date, *I'll only let him get to third base, then I'll make him stop.* Yeah, right. How many times have women made that promise, only to wake up the next morning wondering where they lost their resolve?

The truth is that a good French kiss (a.k.a. "first base") can get your sexual juices flowing like Niagara Falls, a little nipple stimulation ("second base") stimulates a lot more than just your breasts, and letting a man touch your vaginal area ("third base") is simply opening the door wide to a very good possibility of intercourse (or a "home run"). Too bad some of us didn't understand the anatomy of female arousal when we were single. Perhaps we could have maintained healthier boundaries in our dating relationships. But all is not lost. Now that we are married, understanding the "Oh!" behind female sexual arousal can exponentially enhance our sex life and marriage if we are willing to simply take things one base at a time.

For example, your husband asks, "Do you want to have sex?" You check your internal radar and see not even a blip on your sexual screen. You reply, "No, thanks." He goes to bed feeling horny and rejected (not a good combination—ask any man). You go to bed wondering why his sex drive is so much stronger than yours. But if you'll remember the secret of female sexual arousal, you might be happy to get in the game and play at your own pace.

Here's how it works. Instead of replying with a flat-out no, just try going to first base. Tell him, "Nothing's happening down there yet, but I'll bet if you start with paying my lips some attention, we might could fix that!" Feel the warmth of his lips pressing against yours. Listen to how your breathing patterns change, both of you inhaling and exhaling together, and taking in each other's intoxicating aroma. Feel the wetness of his tongue as he explores your lips, then ventures into the crevice of your mouth in search of an identical friend to frolic with. Remember your courtship days, when you felt as if you could let him kiss you for hours, and the cravings those kisses created to feel him touch your yearning body.

When you are ready to go to second base, take his hands and cup them around your breasts. Let him caress your soft skin and massage your body. Soon, his hands will move over and make room for his mouth, as his tongue explorations move from your lips southward. Affirm your readiness by running your fingers through his hair, enjoying the view as he bows down to the breast goddesses. Feel your nipples become more erect than you thought possible, and allow yourself to relax and delightfully indulge in the pleasure of the moment.

Whenever you feel ready, encourage him to go from second base to third, spreading your legs and sending him signals that his wonderful hands are welcome there. Let him manually, visually, and orally explore your private playground, showing him how you'd like to be touched if necessary. Don't feel rushed to reciprocate yet. Just enjoy the pleasure signals your body is sending your brain right now. Let this pleasure nourish your spirit and draw the two of you closer emotionally. Now that you are fully present at third base, home plate doesn't seem so far away, does it?

Before you step outside for some fresh air and a cigarette, here's the moral to this story: *Don't make a judgment call on whether you're ready for a home run before you've even experienced first base.* The natural laws of female sexual arousal usually demand that we take things one step at a time, even after we have a wedding band on our finger. So instead of responding, "No, I'm not in the mood" most of the time as if you are frigid, at least give him a chance to get you in the mood. Otherwise, you shoot down your chances (and his) of enjoying the sexual intimacy that our minds, bodies, hearts, and souls naturally crave.

Once we are primed for some third base and home run action, a few "Oh!" revelations about female orgasm may be helpful in developing our sexual confidence.

The Clitoral "Oh!"

From the time we are toddlers, we're taught, "This is your nose; it is for smelling. This is your tongue; it is for tasting. These are your eyes; they are for seeing." But rarely is a female ever told, "This is your clitoris; it's for having orgasms." Can't envision your mama ever teaching you that? Neither can I. Most of us had to figure it out on our own. Too bad, because I get frequent e-mails from women who, even in their thirties, forties, and fifties, have yet to experience their first "Oh!" moment when it comes to clitoral orgasm. For example, Cindy writes:

I first heard the word *orgasm* when I was in high school, but no one ever really explained it, and I was too embarrassed to ask. I pretended to know all about it. From what I could tell from the movies, it involved some moaning and groaning, and sinking of fingernails into the flesh of your partner's back.

Then I got married, and on our honeymoon night, I moaned, and I groaned, and I sank my nails into my husband's back thinking this would enhance the experience. It must have enhanced it for him, because within seconds he was coming inside me. Then he rolled over and we were done. I was too naive to know what I was missing, so I figured that's as good as it gets.

Fast forward thirteen years and three children later. My husband brings home a gag gift from a white elephant Christmas party at the office. It's a battery-powered, penis-shaped dildo. Not wanting to toss it in the trash can for fear our children would find it, he tucked it into his underwear drawer, and we both forgot about it. Well, *he* forgot about it. I remembered it one day while putting his laundry away, and I decided to see what it felt like. I turned it on and just placed it between my legs. It was too rigid and bulky to feel all that great inside of me, but I noticed that it felt fantastic just resting against me. That's when I discovered a "hot spot" I never knew I had. Although my husband had touched my clitoris with his fingers before, it was usually just briefly, to help me get lubricated. Not enough to really get me going like this thing did. I couldn't believe how great it felt! After only a few minutes, a wave of intense pleasure washed over me, causing every muscle in my body to contract. Then my vaginal muscles began throbbing in a way I had never experienced. It lasted only a few seconds, then my whole body relaxed completely, and I felt like runny oatmeal for the next several minutes.

As I rested there on our bed, I had mixed emotions. On the one hand, I was angry that no one had ever told me that my body was capable of this, especially my husband. On the other hand, I was so excited about my new discovery that thirteen years of faking it out of ignorance didn't seem to matter. I finally had my "Oh!" moment, and I was looking forward to many more real Os.

Cindy's experience isn't uncommon. Many women report that their first orgasm occurs during some form of self-pleasuring experience, whether using a vibrator, sitting near a hot tub or swimming pool jet, or simply using their fingers for clitoral exploration.

However, the goal for the sexually confident wife is to learn how to experience orgasmic pleasure in the presence of her husband rather than in solitary confinement. Remember, as we discussed in Chapter 2, one of the key purposes of sexuality is to pair-bond, not fly solo.

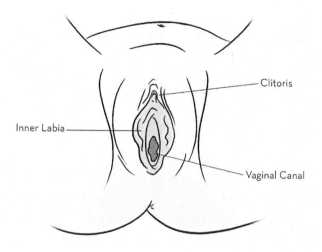

Clitoris

Inner Labia

Vaginal Canal

Designed for Pleasure

Did you know the female clitoris has eight thousand nerve fibers? That's almost twice as many as the male penis! In fact, the clitoris has the highest concentration of nerve fibers in the entire body. What purpose do all of these nerve fibers serve? They exist for no other biological reason than to provide women tremendous sexual pleasure![1]

We'll talk more about self-pleasuring in the context of marriage in Chapter 10, but for now, let's hear from Melissa about her "Oh!" moment.

The G-Spot "Oh!"

In her midforties, Melissa has been married to Doug for twenty-two years. Both reported feeling satisfied in their sex life throughout the majority of their marriage, with the exception of those few difficult months after giving birth to twins. Now that the twins are away at college, they are basking in their empty nest and having more sex than they've had since they were newlyweds. And because practice makes perfect, they've stumbled upon something new, even after all these years of making love.

> While I've always enjoyed intercourse, foreplay is what really gets my motor revving. I've always told my husband that he has magic fingers, as he's never had a problem bringing me to orgasm within a few minutes just by stroking my clitoris. But one night Doug inserted one finger, then two, inside my vaginal canal and stimulated me for longer than he ever has without removing his fingers and moving on to some other pleasurable activity. It seemed like the longer he fingered me, the more relaxed I became. Then all of a sudden, I felt the need to bear down, kind of like when you are delivering a baby. As I did, Doug continued to stimulate me and his hand almost got swept up in a tidal wave of sexual juices flowing out of me! I thought "female ejaculation" was just a term made up by the porn industry to sell more videos, but it's actually possible for a woman to come even more than a man ejaculates!

Melissa is right. The fantastic female body is actually made to experience far more pleasure than most of us ever realize. But with some patience, perseverance, and practice, you can also experience blissful G-spot orgasms (named after Ernest Grafenberg, who called the public's attention to this part of the female anatomy in the 1950s). The G-spot actually refers to the paraurethral glands and nerves, which are located between the urethra and vaginal canal.

Here's a few things you should be aware of when it comes to G-spot orgasms:

- To locate your G-spot, lie on your back. Invite your husband to lie close to you on his side, with one arm cradling your shoulders and one hand between your legs (or however feels comfortable, but physical and emotional closeness are key). Have him insert his middle finger into your vaginal canal with his palm facing the ceiling. Once you are fully relaxed, he should bend his middle finger slightly, forming a soft upward "hook" so that the pad of his finger places slight pressure on the anterior (front) portion of your vaginal canal. As he continues to rub you in this way for some time, your vaginal muscles will eventually begin to bear down, almost pushing his fingers out, but tell him to stay put and keep going until you tell him otherwise.

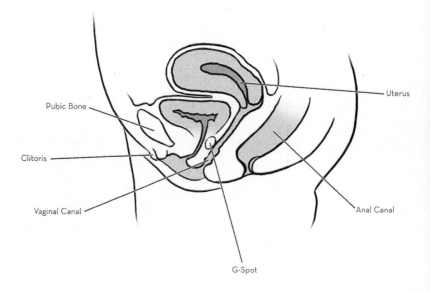

Uterus

Pubic Bone

Clitoris

Vaginal Canal

Anal Canal

G-Spot

- Eventually, a significant amount of fluid will accompany the vaginal contractions, so it is wise to have a layer of protection between you and your sheets or else you'll be sleeping in the wet spot all night, and a towel may not be sufficient. I suggest a small, waterproof crib pad that can easily be thrown in the laundry, or cut a two-foot square piece from an old shower curtain liner or plastic sheet and place that underneath a towel on your bed.

- The expulsion of such a significant amount of fluid could make you think you are wetting the bed. Although the sensation might initially feel similar to urinating, don't worry. The fluid that flows out does not smell or stain like urine. It is clear and odorless, and most men claim that it is tasteless or even slightly sweet to the taste. As a confidence booster, you might empty your bladder just prior to this sexual activity so that when you are relaxed and bearing down, you aren't distracted with concerns about urinating at all.

- Just because you begin to experience this type of orgasm doesn't mean you have to stop! Although multiple orgasms are far more difficult for men, women have the luxury of a much shorter refractory period, which means she can be an orgasmic Energizer bunny and keep going and going if she wants to. A woman's body is capable of experiencing these intense waves of pleasure over and over for several minutes (some report up to half an hour or more). Usually, it's an overwhelming desire for intercourse with her husband that brings these orgasmic waves to an end, as she demands he replaces his fingers with his penis. Some women may even continue experiencing G-spot orgasms during intercourse. You may also find that experiencing a clitoral orgasm through manual or oral stimulation following a G-spot orgasm multiples the pleasure factor exponentially!

In her book *Women: An Intimate Geography,* Natalie Angier insightfully states, "[Some women] never bought Freud's idea of penis envy; who would want a shotgun when you can have a semiautomatic?"[2] ●

- Don't get disappointed or down on yourself if you fail to reach this lofty peak every single time you make love. It's not about the quantity of orgasms you experience but rather the quality of the sexual relationship you and your husband share together.

Perhaps you are thinking that experiencing multiple orgasms would make you a sexually selfish person, or an orgasm hog, or some sort of wild woman that you've never aspired to become. Get over that fear. Most men would give their right arm or left nut for their wives to be this sexually responsive.

You're Worth It

A final "Oh!" worth mentioning is that women simply take longer (sometimes ten times longer) to reach orgasm than men. While he may only need two or three minutes, she usually needs twenty or thirty minutes. Don't feel bad about this, as if it's so much harder on him to perform all that work that you'll just settle for the three minutes. That's ultimately robbing you both, and you'll eventually grow to feel resentful because sex seems to be too much about him and not enough about you. The fact is that most husbands don't want to be perceived as selfish lovers. Sure, it may be a good hand or tongue workout to stimulate you for half an hour or as long as it takes to help you orgasm, but most men really don't mind. After all, the payoff is pretty great—getting to watch his beautiful wife shudder with overwhelming pleasure and experience the big "O" because of how he makes her feel.

If you've never experienced some of these "Oh!" moments, please know that you are not alone. Ten to 15 percent of American women have never experienced any kind of orgasm at all, and only 35 percent of the female population will orgasm during intercourse.[3] We'll talk more about female orgasm in Chapter 13, addressing the question, "What if I need a little help?"

One bit of good news, however, is that 90 percent of orgasmic problems are psychological in nature.[4] In other words, most of the problem isn't between our legs but rather between our ears. The "stinking thinking" we often engage in translates into sexual insecurities, and those insecurities gravitate from our head to our pelvis. By allowing this to happen, we rob ourselves of that which is our birthright as females—sexual pleasure and fulfillment.

For that reason, the entire next section of the book is dedicated to changing the way we think and feel simply by changing the way we behave. As the saying goes, "It's easier to act your way into a new way of feeling than to feel your way into a new way of acting." So if you are ready to act, think, and feel like a sexually confident wife, then let's go behind closed doors.

Part 4

Getting Behind Closed Doors

9

Developing a Girl Scout Mentality

As a frequent conference speaker, I often have the same horrific nightmare. I'm introduced by someone and called out on stage, but soon realize that I have nothing prepared to say. I hem and haw a little bit and try to come up with something worth talking about, then exit stage left when I realize that it's no use. Fortunately, this nightmare has never become a reality because I've learned the importance of that famous Girl Scout motto: *Be prepared!* With the proper preparation, I'm never wanting for confidence as I take the microphone, speak my mind, and share my heart with my audience.

Almost two decades of marriage has also taught me the importance of preparation, not as a speaker but as a sexual human being. You may be thinking, *But sexual encounters should be spontaneous, not rehearsed!* I completely agree. However, women would do themselves a big favor to recognize the importance of a little advance preparation for those spontaneous encounters. Why? Because if we don't feel prepared to entertain his spontaneous sexual advances (for whatever reason), we're far more likely to spurn them. In addition, we're far less likely to initiate spontaneous encounters with our mate if we feel unprepared for a positive sexual experience. Therefore, let's examine what I believe are seven of the most common confidence *busters,* along with seven corresponding confidence *boosters.*

Confidence Buster #1: Burning the Candle at Both Ends

Our society places such value on busyness. It seems as if our identity as human beings comes not from who we are as people but from what we do with our time. The underlying sentiment is that the busier you are, the more important you are, and the more important you are, the more valuable you must be. Take a look at many women's day planners, and their daily agenda looks something like this:

7:30 a.m.	Pack kids' lunches and get them off to school.
7:45 a.m.	Deliver dog to vet and drop off car at shop.
8:30 a.m.	Work an eight-hour day, running errands at lunch.
6:00 p.m.	Help the kids with homework.
7:00 p.m.	Make dinner and do dishes.
8:00 p.m.	Fold and put away laundry.
8:30 p.m.	Bake and frost cupcakes for tomorrow's soccer practice.
9:00 p.m.	Open mail, pay bills, return phone calls and e-mails.
9:30 p.m.	Pack briefcase and set out everyone's clothes for the next day.
10:00 p.m.	Fall into bed exhausted!

Notice something missing? When does she have time for herself? When does she have time for her husband? Where will she ever muster the energy for sexual intimacy to enhance their marriage or satisfy their personal needs for pleasure and connection? While many individuals wear their busyness like a badge of honor, realize that there's no Brownie badge for being a burned-out woman. And when we choose to burn the candle at both ends, burnout is inevitable. Don't allow busyness to rob you or your marriage. Develop a Girl Scout mentality and prepare yourself to reserve some energy for what's really most important to you.

Confidence Booster #1: Reserving Energy for Life's Priorities

Chances are, if someone asked you who the most important people in your life are, you'd say your husband and children. And while our family certainly has domestic needs that we often have to make a priority in our day, there's nothing your family needs more than for Mom and Dad to have a healthy relationship and be happy with each other.

If your days and weeks are incredibly full, relying on spontaneity for your sexual encounters may require as much wishful thinking as winning the lottery. Be intentional and schedule a little quality time together if necessary. With a little bit of energy dedicated in the right direction, fifteen to thirty minutes at least two or three times each week can feel like an emotional and sexual feast! Are you an early bird? Then set your alarm fifteen minutes early and plan on some sunrise fun in the sheets! Or maybe a little late-afternoon delight while the kids are playing outside or watching cartoons is your prime time for sexual play! If you're more of a night owl, that's okay, but be careful to go to bed early enough to enjoy some real quality time together before you run out of gas and become a bleary-eyed zombie.

Once you settle on the best time for your romantic rendezvous, make everything else work around that commitment. Think of creative ways of saving time and energy for these intimate times together. For example, we don't watch much television during the week, because it's usually a big time-waster. I also save time and energy by doubling or tripling my recipes whenever possible, freezing the extra batch or two so that my dinner preparation time can be slashed on future nights, giving me more time with Greg. We also take turns preparing dinner, or we have an occasional "fend for yourself" night where everyone eats whatever they are willing to fix for themselves. Obviously, my goal in life isn't to be the next Martha Stewart. My goal is to be the best Shannon Ethridge I can be, which requires that I cater to other things besides nightly gourmet meals with all of the trimmings.

Also, consider how your children can help free you up to be a more sexually confident and connected wife. Once my children turned ten years old, they had a daily chore and became responsible for their own laundry. This gave them a sense of pride and accomplishment, while it let me reclaim that time and energy.

Confidence Buster #2: Neglecting Personal Hygiene

Even if you reserve plenty of time and energy for intimate sexual encounters, you may discover a lack of sexual interest on your husband's part if you fail to make personal hygiene a priority as well. Foul odors and tastes will quickly rob *both* a husband and wife of their sexual confidence, as was evidenced in my conversation with Kyle and Emily. Married eight months, Emily was exasperated by her husband's "sexual selfishness" and lack of interest in performing oral sex in order to bring her to orgasm. "I'm happy to give him head practically every time, yet all he ever thinks about is himself. He'll only touch me enough to get me wet, but once he's done getting his own jollies, he's done," Emily complained. After several such attacks, Kyle couldn't take the criticism any longer and finally spoke the truth. "I don't mind giving oral sex! In fact, I enjoy it, but not when you smell bad!" he exploded. I was embarrassed for Emily, but glad the root of the issue was finally being exposed so that it could be remedied.

Upon further questioning, I discovered that Emily's mother had given her the impression that an "earthy" smell was natural and that douches and deodorants were dangerous to the sensitive vaginal region. This is only partially true, so let's look at our next confidence booster to get the whole truth.

Confidence Booster #2: Showering and Shaving

You may have heard Dr. Mehmet Oz on the *Oprah* show talking about how the "va-jay-jay" (as Oprah calls it) is a "self-cleaning oven," but even the best self-cleaning oven requires that you manually clean the front of the oven door!

Granted, the *vaginal canal* (where the penis is inserted and where a baby exits the womb) is a self-cleaning oven, and to use a douche too often can upset your pH balance and wash away good, disease-fighting bacteria. Most doctors advise women not to use a douche at all for this reason. However, for your husband to get to the vaginal canal, he must encounter the labia, and that *is not a self-cleaning area.* In fact, just like every other crack and crevice in your body, it is a breeding ground for odor-causing bacteria. Spraying feminine deodorants on this area may mask foul smells, but it only covers them up and may leave an unpleasant taste for your husband to have to deal with.

So if a woman shouldn't douche and deodorants are insufficient, what should she do? There are special products such as Summer's Eve Intimate Cleanser made to be used just like soap on a woman's vaginal area. It isn't inserted into the vaginal canal, but rather massaged between your outer labia majora and inner labia minora to wash away foul odors and leave you feeling fresh and confident. Some types of intimate cleansers are especially made for sensitive skin, but if you find that you break out as a result of using such products, you can still sit in a warm tub of water and use a washcloth to wipe your vaginal area clean.

This type of cleansing is especially important following your menstrual cycle, but can actually be done every day if you choose, which will certainly provide a sense of sexual confidence every time your husband spontaneously gets all touchy-feely! You won't have to kill the moment by responding to his advances, "Oh, wait, I'm not clean right now! Wait until later!" Later may or may not happen.

In addition to cleansing your vaginal area, an occasional intimate shave may also be an effort that your husband really appreciates. After all, oral sex can't be as pleasant for either one of you when he's having to work around a mouthful of pubic hair. My best recommendation is to invite your husband to perform this service for you while you lie cleansed and bare on a towel. Assuming he'll take things slow and be sensitive, he's got the best visual view of what should be snipped and trimmed away and what should remain out of harm's way.

Be aware that if you decide to go for the naked-as-the-day-you-were-born shave, it's going to make for some fantastic sensations during lovemaking for about the first twenty-four hours. Beyond that, you may find yourself with a very itchy rash as the hair grows back. For that reason, I recommend just a really close trim, using a barber's comb and clippers for a close "burr haircut." It lasts a good while, there's no itchy rash involved, and it still makes for a great view.

Of course, there's also the Brazilian bikini wax if you're game, which produces an incredibly smooth hair-free surface on the outer labia and anus. He can indulge physically and visually for weeks before the hair grows back, and you'll be super-sensitive to his every touch (in a good way). Yes, there's a few seconds of pain associated with this procedure, but most women report that the sexual confidence it creates is well worth the effort!

Confidence Buster #3: Wearing Granny Panties

Speaking of views, do you realize that the underwear you choose can either make or break your sexual confidence? As you undress in your husband's presence, do you feel like catching his eye and flaunting your beautiful body, or running and hiding behind your fuzzy robe?

I know, I know. You may be thinking, *But I like my underwear to be extremely comfortable! And I don't want any panty lines showing through my pants!* So you choose to wear great big white granny panties to ensure complete comfort and coverage. Maybe your walk on the wild side includes wearing colored granny panties on special days. Well, guess what? Men don't fantasize about having sex with their granny, and you don't have to wear granny panties to get an incredibly comfortable fit!

Confidence Booster #3: Wearing Comfortable, Sexy Lingerie

I'm a big advocate of throwing all of your granny panties away since discovering Jockey's No Panty Line Promise line of lingerie (www.jockey.com). Their panties come in a variety of shapes and styles, but my favorite is the basic low-rise bikini. Made of a silky stretch nylon with gentle elastic, they really do stay in place so you don't have to tug at them all the time to keep them out of your crack. They provide a smooth foundation for a sexy silhouette underneath any clothes. And best of all, they make you look (and feel) sexy as all get-out! Combine a black pair of Jockey No Panty Line Promise bikinis with a satiny push-up bra, and your husband's going to chase you down the hallway thinking you look good enough to eat.

When shopping for lingerie, comfort and coverage are important, but so is confidence in the way you look. If you don't like the way you look in your lingerie, you're going to assume that your husband doesn't like the way you look, either. The same goes for pajamas (if you must wear them at all). Climb into bed looking frumpy, and you're going to feel frumpy. There's too many cute and comfy camis and shorts and nighties these days to go to bed looking like your grandma! Don't be afraid to shop for something comfy *and* sexy!

Confidence Buster #4: Fearing Intrusive Children

Okay, so you've carved out some special time for your man, you've showered and shaved that morning, and you've been wearing your comfortable, sexy underwear all day. You're finally ready for some adult connection time now that the dishes are done. But there's one big thing holding you back—that forty-pound preschooler banging at your bedroom door, screaming, *"Mom-meeeeee!* What are you doing in there? Open the door!"

Probably every mother has experienced the overwhelming fear of "What if the kids walk in?" during intimate moments together. While it's good to be a vigilant parent, it's not good to be a sexually frustrated vigilant parent, so let's talk about the right to our own time outs.

Confidence Booster #4: Claiming a Parental "Time Out"

Train your children early in life that mommies and daddies need their special time together and that it's very inconsiderate to disturb them during these times. To make sure you get that special time, consider installing some sort of lock or hook-and-eye latch on your bedroom door to prevent any unwelcome surprises.

As soon as our children were old enough to comprehend, we explained, "Erin, you know how much fun it is to have Mommy all to yourself to play and all of her attention is on you and no one else? And other times, it's fun to have Daddy all to yourself for some special playtime? Well, there are times when Mommy and Daddy want to have each other all to ourselves. Do you think you can watch this thirty-minute Barney tape without knocking on Mommy and Daddy's bedroom door? If so, there'll be a reward at the end of the movie." This was easy-breezy with our compliant daughter. But our mischievous son was more resistant to the idea. He tried to insist on joining our private little party, so we had to create additional rules and incentives. "If you knock and we say we'll be out in a minute, you have to go read a book or play by yourself. If you keep knocking, you'll be sent to bed early tonight." Of course, he knocked for some reason every time we closed the door, so we made a new rule. "You're not allowed to disturb us unless there is blood or vomit!" we declared. He eventually got the idea.

This may sound a little cruel, but it actually is a very healthy thing for children to learn boundaries and to understand that husbands and wives need private time alone together. One day we walked out of our bedroom after about thirty minutes of afternoon delight, and twelve-year-old Matthew sheepishly grinned and proclaimed, "I know what you guys were doing in there!" We just smiled back with a wink. Then I asked, "And when you have your own wife someday, are you going to look forward to your private times alone together?" He snickered and replied, "Uh-huh! But not yet!"

Or maybe it's not as much what's going on outside your bedroom as what's going on inside your bedroom that kills your sexual confidence . . .

Confidence Buster #5: Getting Sidetracked by Surroundings

You wouldn't think that something as tiny and frail as a cobweb could derail a steamy sexual experience, but I know from experience that it can! We live in a log cabin made out of rough-cut cedar trees, which means that dusting the inside walls can give you major splinters. Although the cabin is a man's paradise, I had to grow to appreciate the rusticity of the house and learn to live with the "natural" look, including the occasional hard-to-reach cobweb on the vaulted ceiling and support beams. One day I complained, "I'm sorry, but it's really hard to concentrate when I'm staring up at a ceiling full of cobwebs!" I hoped Greg would take the hint, get the extra-tall ladder from outside, and scale up to the rafters to rid me of the distraction. Instead, he jokingly replied, "Then you get on top and I'll stare up at it!" Until those cobwebs came down, all future sexual encounters were going to be a chore for me, I could tell.

What distracts you during sex? Is it the peeling wallpaper? The mound of laundry on the floor? The stacks of books and papers on the bedside table? The icky color you picked out in completely different lighting at the paint store? Regardless of what it is, make it a priority to fix it, girlfriend!

Confidence Booster #5: Creating a Peaceful Private Sanctuary

Fortunately, we've added on to our log cabin, creating a whole master level that I've been able to decorate however I want. Now my son stares up at a vaulted log ceiling (and cobwebs) in our old room and I get to stare at my own peaceful, private sanctuary. Tucked into the branches of a towering oak tree with an entire wall of windows for a natural view of the great outdoors, with a color palette of soothing mossy greens and rich browns, our third-floor master bedroom has a tree house feel, just as we wanted. We kept the furnishings simple, with a comfy king-size bed, padded headboard, satiny comforter, two small nightstands and lamps, and two overstuffed swivel chairs with a matching ottoman where we can play footsie during late-night conversations. We adorned one wall with three sconces, allowing us to illuminate the room with thirty glowing tealight candles and fill the air with a yummy vanilla smell. My bedroom is now a great aphrodisiac rather than a distraction.

Perhaps remodeling and creating a whole new master bedroom isn't a possibility, but there are guidelines that you can implement to ensure that your bedroom resembles a sanctuary more than an insane asylum. First, establish the room's purpose. It's exclusively for resting and relaxing, and enjoying good sleep and great sex. So get rid of anything that doesn't fit that purpose. Don't try to make your bedroom part office. It only reminds you of all the work you should be doing at any given moment. Don't let the kids bring their toys in your room. That's what their rooms and family rooms are for. Don't let your bedroom become the laundry zone, or the scrapbooking zone, or any other zone that doesn't enhance your marital intimacy and fuel a sense of sexual confidence in you. If there's too much clutter in your room, declutter it. If the wallpaper bugs you, change it. If the color isn't soothing and sensual, paint it. If the noise from neighbors up above or traffic down below bothers you, put on a mood-enhancing CD to drown out distractions. No matter what it takes, create a place where you want to let your hair down, get comfy, and get connected with your mate.

Confidence Buster #6: Letting the Well Run Dry

Once you create a room full of romantic ambience, chances are that things are going to get a little hotter in there. And when things get hot, women should be getting wet. It's how our bodies are designed. When a woman sees, hears, smells, tastes, or feels something that arouses her sexual senses, her vaginal canal (or "private well") automatically lubricates. However, such isn't always the case, and it can certainly rob a woman of pleasure and sexual confidence when her private well runs dry, not to mention what this does to her husband's pleasure and confidence.

Sometimes vaginal dryness occurs due to hormonal changes, such as after she's had a baby, or as she experiences menopausal symptoms. Other times, it's simply a matter of her sexual juices running low before the final flow of orgasmic release. Regardless of the reason, there are plenty of reliable cures.

Confidence Booster #6: Keeping Lotions and Potions Nearby

A week before my wedding, a dear older friend asked if she could take me out for a premarital chat over breakfast. I'll never forget the sweetness on her face when she finished her pancakes, put down her fork, and insisted, "Now, Shannon, the most important thing you need to remember to pack for your honeymoon is K-Y Jelly!"

Good thing she shared this little tidbit with me, because I'd have been up a sexual creek without a paddle (or lubrication) without her sage advice. Or I might have made the mistake that many naive couples have made and used Vaseline instead. Vaseline will solve the dryness problem, but it will also form a moisture barrier that can cause a vaginal infection, so save the Vaseline for your baby's butt and invest in a female lubricant designed for sexual purposes. While K-Y Jelly is considered the old standby and used in many hospitals (for reasons other than sex, obviously!), there are some newer personal lubricants that also come highly recommended, such as Astroglide and Wet. Tuck a bottle into your nightstand drawer for easy reach when needed. Don't worry about the kids finding it. If they do, they'll eventually put two and two together that the marriage bed is a happening kind of place! And that's not such a bad thing when you consider the alternatives. (We'll talk more about instilling sexual values in children in the last chapter.)

Of course, when your husband discovers that you are keeping these magical lotions and potions within arm's reach, he may reach over for some loving more often than before. That's why the final confidence buster I'd like you to avoid is feeling like a piece of meat.

Confidence Buster #7: Feeling Like a Piece of Meat

When Cheryl and Dan first married, they had sex several times per week. As kids, careers, and household responsibilities demanded more and more of their time and energy, their sex life dwindled down to once every week or two, and Cheryl was actually fine with that. But Dan grew more disgruntled and frustrated over Cheryl's lack of attention to his sexual needs. His nightly tactic was to try to initiate sex with his wife fully expecting rejection, then using her negative response as justification for his next action—to sneak down to his office to peep at porn online and take sexual matters into his own hands. After months of this routine, however, he felt guilty about the use of pornography and committed to break the habit. He confessed to his wife and asked if she'd please be more open to his sexual advances.

The first night Dan approached her, she was surprisingly compliant because she felt bad about how long it had been since they'd had sex. A few nights later, they even had sex again when Cheryl initiated this time. But soon, Cheryl felt that because Dan was initiating more often than she cared for, he was being greedy to expect her to pick up the sexual pace in their relationship. "Why are you pawing on me so often lately? Am I just a piece of meat to you?" she asked Dan one night, piercing his heart and deflating his sexual desire for her.

If you've ever shared Cheryl's sentiment and felt like nothing more than an outlet for his sexual tension, perhaps it's time to consider the final intimacy booster . . .

Confidence Booster #7: Feeling Like a Sexual Goddess

If you're like me, no one ever prepared you for the fact that there's often a noticeable difference between the male sex drive and the female sex drive. Male hormones race around in his body faster than a Nascar racer on his final lap, whereas female hormones just kind of meander around in our bodies like a lovely horse-drawn carriage clopping through a downtown square. We can feel rather put out or imposed upon when he revs up his engines and comes speeding in our direction to satisfy his sexual appetite. But if we're going to develop a Girl Scout mentality, we'll prepare ourselves for these frequent and often unexpected sexual inquiries. We'll understand that we're far more than a pit stop on his road to sexual release. We're more than a piece of meat to this hungry lion. We're a sexual goddess that he bows down to, hoping to discover a level of satisfaction and pleasure that he's not allowed to enjoy with any other woman.

I don't intend to be irreverent or idolatrous here. I'm not telling you to lord it over him that you've got some sort of power over him, but the reality is that you do. If you don't cook for him, he can go to McDonald's. If you don't launder his shirts, he can drop them off at the cleaners. If you don't keep house for him, he can hire a maid. But if you won't provide an inviting outlet for his sexual release, where can he go? What can he do?

We don't want to know the answer to that question. We want to embrace our role as his sexual goddess—the woman he can bring his deepest, most intimately felt needs to and trust that she'll cure whatever ails him. She'll remove the tension from his body as often as necessary. She'll put a smile on his face over and over. She'll put a song in his heart, a song that says, "I love having a sexually confident wife!"

> "Sex is part of nature. I go along with nature."
> —*Marilyn Monroe, actress*

I'm not telling you to abandon your own sexual and emotional needs in order to cater to his. Tend to your own needs and desires so that it's a mutually beneficial encounter. Ask him to take you out to dinner, and rub his leg with your foot underneath the table. Invite him to take a bubble bath with you and scrub your back. Wrap your loving arms around him and pray for him, praising him for all that he is and does for you, and listen intently as he does the same for you.

Remember that being his sex partner isn't meant to be a burden. It's meant to be a blessing, not just to him but to both of you. You're his beloved wife. You're his most intimate friend. You're his sex goddess. He doesn't want to just wipe his feet on any sexual doormat. He wants to feast at a table of sexual delights—*your* table of sexual delights. So set the table and invite him to come hungry!

A Quick Refresher Course

If you're ready to develop a Girl Scout mentality and make sure you are prepared to enjoy the most phenomenal sex life possible, let's recap these confidence busters and confidence boosters, shall we?

Sexual Confidence Busters	Sexual Confidence Boosters
1. Burning the Candle at Both Ends	1. Reserving Energy for Life's Priorities

2. Neglecting Personal Hygiene	2. Showering and Shaving
3. Wearing Granny Panties	3. Wearing Comfortable, Sexy Lingerie
4. Fearing Intrusive Children	4. Claiming a Parental "Time Out"
5. Getting Sidetracked by Surroundings	5. Creating a Peaceful Private Sanctuary
6. Letting the Well Run Dry	6. Keeping Lotions and Potions Nearby
7. Feeling Like a Piece of Meat	7. Feeling Like a Sexual Goddess

Of course, there are times when the only things required to pre-pare for a fantastic sexual experience is pure passion and an amo-rous attitude. For example, the other night the kids were both away and Greg and I were walking around our hundred-acre plot of land by ourselves. I spotted the trampoline nestled among several pine trees and gravitated over to it, leading Greg by the hand into this private haven. Even though I had a to-do list a mile long awaiting me inside, I decided there was nothing more important than surpris-ing Greg's socks off, as well as all other articles of clothing. But I had exercised hard that day and was all sweaty and gross. I was still wearing my grungy cycling shorts and T-shirt, a far cry from sexy bikini underwear or a slinky nightie, but I figured I'd better seize my moment for shock value.

Unaware of my plan, Greg sat down in a lawn chair beside the trampoline as I hopped on and began jumping. His eyes began to twinkle when he figured out what I had in mind as I began stripping down piece by piece. When he climbed up and joined me, I offered to run inside, shower, shave, put on something a little sexier, and rejoin him on the trampoline momentarily, but we couldn't stop kissing, or hugging, or touching. We didn't stop. We simply kept going until we collapsed under the pine trees, breathless and sweatier than ever.

I laughed afterward, explaining that I was currently writing a chapter on developing a Girl Scout mentality and always being prepared for a spontaneous sexual encounter but that I just failed my own course. Greg replied, "A sexually confident wife certainly needs a 'Girl Scout' mentality at times. Other times she just needs a 'Nike' mentality: *Just do it!*"

Greg's right. Just do it, girlfriend. Prepare however you can, do it as often as you can, and enjoy every minute of it!

10

Tantalizing Sexual Techniques

When you hear the term *missionary position,* what comes to mind? If the *position* part of the term strikes you, you most likely envision a couple facing each other horizontally and having intercourse while the man is on top. If the *missionary* part of the term strikes you, perhaps you envision devout religious people spreading the myth that this form of sexual intercourse is the only acceptable one in God's eyes. Or perhaps the term evokes completely different images altogether for whatever reason. Maybe this is one of your favorite sexual positions, and your husband's, too. If so, don't let me discourage you from enjoying it! However, in the spirit of maximizing sexual fulfillment in your marriage, I want to challenge you to think outside the missionary box.

Do you want to know what comes to my mind when I hear the term *missionary position*? Honestly, I think of lazy women and bored men.

I'm not saying this position can't be fun and pleasurable, but let's be honest. Oftentimes it's used for lack of creativity or energy. At the end of the day, he's feeling frisky and she's feeling exhausted. He attempts to initiate. She grimaces on the inside but succumbs to his advances only if he's willing to do the work. With the lights off and the covers up, she spreads her legs, he rolls over to mount, and wham, bam, thank you, ma'am, we have intercourse. But where's the passion? The energy and excitement? The playful titillation?

Maybe I'm overdramatizing just a bit, but if we're honest, this is often how our sexual relationship plays itself out. All of the fun, frivolity, and fulfillment get lost in our sexual laziness and relational apathy. But it doesn't have to be that way. We can have extremely rewarding sexual experiences if we're willing to move beyond the missionary position and incorporate some more tantalizing sexual techniques into our repertoire—techniques that we can implement both inside and outside the bedroom.

"Easy sex, where a woman lies on a bed and you get on top of her, isn't very interesting. I'm a man, I like a struggle, a conquest. I just happen to like being the loser, and then made to satisfy the female winner."
—*Eric Stanton, erotic cartoonist*

If you're not sure where to begin, let's start with some of the basics, focusing on what turns him on most and brings you great pleasure in the process.

I asked my husband to complete this sentence in at least five different ways:

"What really gets me going sexually is . . ."

Since he's a typical red-blooded American male, I believe his honest responses speak for most men:

1. When you give me that "I want you" smile.
2. When you kiss me—I mean *really* kiss me.
3. When you reveal parts or all of your body for my viewing pleasure.
4. When you show me you're into it by initiating creative sexual positions.
5. When you touch me in ways that you know send me through the roof!

Let's explore these five responses and imagine how we can incorporate a few more tantalizing sexual techniques into our everyday existence, enhancing our sexual confidence and our husband's confidence as well.

"Whenever I see your smiling face, I have to smile myself..." (James Taylor, 1977)

Remembering back to when we were teenage girls, what was one of the first signs we looked for to discern if a guy really liked us? His smile. We could pass him in the hallway hundreds of times or talk to him throughout our lunch period, but until he started smiling directly at us, we really weren't sure of his feelings. His sweet smile seemed to announce, "Hey, I think you're great! You make me happy! I like being with you!" And most likely, your smile said the same thing to him.

Your husband is basically a teenage boy trapped in a grown man's body. He still needs discernible signs that you like him, that you love him, and that you crave him sexually. And what better way to remind him of those things than to simply look at him and smile frequently?

Maybe you are thinking, *But I need to have a reason to smile!* Funny, we never needed a reason as a giddy teenage girl. It just came naturally. What's happened to that smile now that we're all grown up? We've bought the lie that our happiness comes from external sources, and we wait for someone or something to paint a smile on our face rather than reach inside for reasons to smile.

But what if I told you that smiling *first* can produce genuine happiness as a result? It's true! Studies indicate that it is not as much that our facial expressions are reflections of our feelings as it is that our feelings are largely reflections of the facial expressions we wear.[1] In other words, the more you smile, the happier you feel. And the more you shoot him a sexy smile, the sexier you'll feel!

How much time and energy is required to offer a smile? Almost none. But how far could it go in developing a sense of sexual confidence and rapport between you and your husband? A long, long way.

"Your kiss is on my list of the best things in life!"
(Darryl Hall and John Oates, 1980)

Do you want my personal translation of Greg's second response, "When you kiss me—I mean *really* kiss me"? He was saying, "I don't just want a peck in passing, or a 'Have a great day!' kiss at the door. I want one of your passion-filled kisses—one that leaves me weak in the knees and feeling like a real man!"

There's something very magical about a kiss. It's the most basic element in any love story we've ever read or watched—a moment when sparks fly and hearts soar in celebration of mutual attraction.

Don't you remember longing for some special guy to kiss you? Or how much we daydreamed about the wonderful kiss we'd receive from our husband at the altar? Or the kind of wild, indulgent kisses we'd enjoy with reckless abandon on our honeymoon? Yeah. Wonderful, wet "I want you now!" kisses.

While the desire to be kissed can be temporarily satisfied, does the longing to have someone in our lives who *wants* to kiss us ever disappear? I think not. This is true for your husband as well. He doesn't need just an occasional peck on the cheek or "mother" kiss that says, "I love you, honey." He craves a deeply sensual kiss that passionately screams, "I'm deliriously turned on by you, sir!"

"Her kisses left something to be desired—the rest of her."
    —*Anonymous*

Maybe you're thinking that you've lost your appetite for such kisses because you don't necessarily like the way your husband does it. Well, you're only as good as the person you are with, and if he doesn't kiss all that great in your opinion, it's because you haven't taught him what you like! Perhaps his technique is too sloppy, or too stiff, or too wet, or maybe it's his breath that leaves something to be desired. It's okay to communicate your preferences, as long as you do it carefully and constructively. "I hate the way you kiss!" or "Why can't you kiss me more like so-and-so?" would *not* be the best way to approach the topic. Instead, try something like, "I love it when you kiss me, but if you would try not to salivate quite as much, I'd want to kiss you even more often," or "Fresh-breath kisses really turn me on."

If your displeasure is a matter of how he moves his lips and tongue when he kisses you, try this experiment. Tell him you are going to kiss him and you want him to directly imitate only what you are do-ing, exactly the way you are doing it—same movement, same pres-sure, same intensity, and so on. Then model the exact kiss that would sweep you off your feet so that he'll know how you like to be kissed. Offer him the same experience so that you're in the learning seat. He may enjoy a completely different kind of kiss, so be cooperative and play by both sets of kissing rules on occasion.

Finally, don't be stingy with sensual kisses, reserving them strictly as immediate foreplay to sexual activity. Like Clark Gable said to Scarlett O'Hara in *Gone With the Wind*, "You need to be kissed, and often, and by someone who knows how!" Both you and your hus-band need to be kissed often. I encourage couples to kiss several times throughout the day, but at least once each day for a minimum of ten to fifteen seconds. This is easier than you think. Stop him in the hallway and press your soft lips against his for no reason at all. Meet him in the backyard while he's barbecuing just to plant a big juicy one on him. Step into his office, close the door, and kiss him in such a way that he'll be blushing next time he faces his coworkers. And that kiss will most likely leave him wanting more, so let's move on to Greg's third response.

"Baby what a big surprise, right before my very eyes . . ."
(Chicago, 1977)

In case you haven't figured it out already, men have two small round organs that kick their sex drive into high gear. You might think they're located in his pants, but the ones I'm referring to are actually in his head. A man's eyeballs are all that he needs to get his motor running! Are you adding fuel to his visual tank, or expecting him to run on empty much of the time? Be honest. Imagine the past forty-eight hours. How have you dressed and acted around him? Has he had good opportunities to drink your sexy body in through his eyeballs? Or does your hiding behind frumpy clothes leave his engine running idle? Or worse, does your low self-esteem leave him feeling overwhelmingly tempted to look at images of other, less inhibited women?

Let's be real, girlfriends. There's nothing sexy about an inhibited woman. For a man, it's all about exhibition, not inhibition! Their fascination with female exhibitionism is why porn magazines, movies, and websites are so popular with the male species. In pornographic images, you never see women hiding themselves in shame, only women revealing themselves brazenly.

While it is never a wife's fault that her husband turns to pornography rather than to her for sexual gratification, we do possess the power to lessen his desire for it. How? By embracing a sexually confident attitude about our body and giving him all of the visual gratification he desires. In other words, leave the lights on! Throw the covers off! Hiding under blankets in the dark can be fun on occasion, but it's far more visually stimulating and sensually intimate for a couple to make love in full view of each other.

Because one of a man's greatest sexual needs is to gaze upon his wife's scantily clad or nude body, consider these eye-popping, tantalizing techniques to stimulate him visually:

1. *Leave the robe in the closet.* In public parts of the house, by all means, be modest in case one of the kids walks into the room or the UPS deliveryman glances through the window on his way to the front porch. But in the privacy of your own master bedroom and bathroom, why do you need a robe? It just hides what your husband is really eager to experience—an extended glimpse of your beautiful body. Get comfortable in nothing but your bare

skin or sexy underwear, and assure him that he can be comfortable indulging in a long, hard stare whenever he wants one.

2. *Dance or strip for him!* Make getting naked in front of your husband a ritual at your house, entertaining him with an eyeful of erotic movements. For the really adventurous, there are pole-dancing classes where you can learn to prance like the pros. For the moderately adventurous, try an online class or DVD on belly dancing. Carmen Electra's *Striptease Aerobics* not only teaches you all sorts of sexy dancing techniques such as the lap dance but also gives you a great workout, which only enhances your sexual confidence. Double score! If these ideas aren't for you, just try getting his attention by walking toward him while taking off one piece of clothing at a time such that by the time you arrive in his arms, there's nothing hindering him from caressing any part of your body that he desires. Another fun option is to initiate an old-fashioned game of strip poker! You might enjoy it so much that you decide to keep a deck of cards in your nightstand drawer for future use.

3. *Make your own movies!* At a recent conference, one woman wrote a question on a piece of paper and handed it to me privately. I felt it was such a valuable question that it deserved to be shared with everyone, so I read it aloud from the stage. "Is it okay for a married couple to make their own private erotic movies using their own digital camera?"

My answer? Heck yes, it is! And why not? Don't hesitate to set up a tripod in the corner of the room and embrace your role as the sexy star of this show! Strike a pose and invite your husband to take a few up-close-and-personal still shots. View the pictures and movies together to add some excitement to your lovemaking. Just make sure you delete them all before loaning your camera to your teenager.

If you simply can't picture yourself engaging in these exhibition-istic activities because of your feelings about your body, I encourage you to return to Chapter 7 for a refresher course on befriending the body image bear!

Once you've got your husband visually stimulated beyond belief, you're ready to fulfill one of his wildest fantasies—to be pursued by a hot babe who wants his body like crazy!

> *"If you want my body and you think I'm sexy,*
> *Come on, honey, tell me so!"* (Rod Stewart, 1978)

Returning to our opening conversation about the missionary posi-tion, a woman lying flat on her back with legs spread in dread of what's coming next, most likely *isn't* what your husband fantasizes about. Chances are, he wants to be pursued sexually! He wants you to reach out to him at random moments and communicate, whether verbally or through body language, "You've got something I want!" So what better way to affirm his sexual desirability *and* to maximize his viewing pleasure than getting on top for a pleasure ride?

The woman-on-top position can work a number of ways, but just to get your imagination started, here are three ideas to consider:

- *Pony-style*: With your husband lying flat on his back, mount him while supporting your weight on your knees. Benefits of this position include your being able to grace his lips with one of those wonderful wet kisses we just talked about, his being able to stare at your lovely breasts in motion, your setting the sexual pace according to what you find most pleasurable (remember, your pleasure is important to him as well as his own), and his ability to touch your buttocks, breasts, and clitoris.

- *Froggie-style*: Engage in this position in the same way you would the pony position, but rather than resting on your knees, bend your knees and squat over him, balancing your weight with your feet on the bed and your buttocks on his thighs. The added benefit of this position is his ability to get a much clearer view of his penis going back and forth into your vagina, which is a real turn-on for him. You can also put pillows behind you so that you can lean back, giving him an even clearer view, and giving you more G-spot stimulation.

- *Doggie-style*: While most envision doggie-style involving the man on his knees, you can do a modified version with your husband flat on his back and you riding him pony style while facing his feet instead. Benefits? Again, you set the pace for what's pleasurable for you, and he gets the absolute best rear view possible!

If being on top doesn't do that much for you, or if your husband prefers to be on top so that he can exercise more control, or if you're just looking to add variety to your repertoire, there are several ways you can vary the missionary position to be more exciting, playful, and/or visually stimulating. Here's a few ideas in that direction:

- *Living on the Edge*: While lying on your back, slide down to the bottom of the bed such that your rear end is resting on the edge. Invite your husband to stand or kneel at the foot of the bed (according to how high your bed is) and make love to you while in this position. If you have a dresser or bench near the foot of the bed, you could rest your feet on it for support, or you could raise your legs in the air before he enters you such that your knees are either draped over his shoulders or wrapped around his waist.

- *Floating Fun*: In a large whirlpool bathtub such as what you'll find in nicer hotel rooms, float on your back with your legs spread wide, or rest your head on a bath pillow and perch your feet on the sides of the tub. Invite your husband to penetrate you while kneeling in the water, using a submerged towel to cushion his knees.

- *Tight Squeeze*: While in the standard missionary position, consider closing your legs while his penis is still inside your vagina. You'll need to tuck your bottom down and your pelvis up to maintain penetration, but by closing your thighs rather than leaving them apart, your husband's penis will get a tight squeeze that he won't soon forget! In fact, you can add to his sexual pleasure in this way in any position simply by placing your fingers around your external vaginal lips and giving the base of his penis a gentle squeeze. Of course, he may not remain inside you very long when you try this technique, as it has a tendency to send him toward the finish line with great speed!

In addition to initiating various sexual positions to express your exhibitionism and playfulness, there are also some special "hot spots" that you can touch or techniques you can use that will really launch his rocket!

"Do that to me one more time." (Captain and Tennille, 1979)

The male penis is a mystery to most women, because we've never had one. But if you ask your husband where his most sensitive hot spots are, chances are he'd say three places: the tip of his penis (the mushroom-shaped area around the rim of the circumcised penis, or the first one or two inches of the uncircumcised penis), the perineum (the prostate area, between the scrotum and the anus), and the nipples (yes, men like nipple stimulation, too). So let's talk about a few positions or sexual activities that are sure to heighten his pleasure:

- *Scissor Sex*: Begin with the wife lying flat on her back. The husband lies on his right side directly to the left of his wife such that they are facing each other at a 90-degree angle. She drapes her left leg over his body such that her buttocks are pressed against his pelvis area, allowing deep vaginal penetration with his penis. This position is great because both husband and wife get to relax comfortably either on their back or their side, your clitoris is easily within his reach, both partners' nipples are easily accessible, and his perineum can easily be massaged either with your hand or with your thigh by pressing your leg into his crotch as he moves in and out of your vagina. Feel free to use some sort of lotion or lubricant for an added sense of pleasure!

- *Lend a Helping Hand*: If you and your husband are within the same height range, try standing in front of him and bending over as if you are touching your toes. Allow his penis to enter your vagina from behind, then reach through your own thighs and massage his perineum as he is thrusting. Again, a little lubricant or lotion on your fingertips will go a long way toward sending him over the edge while in this position!

- *Rub-a-Dub-Dub Sex*: There's nothing more delightful than a tub for two, whether that's a private hot tub or your personal bathtub. This tantalizing sexual technique can also be done in the shower if you have a bench for him to sit on. Encourage him to have a seat on the inside edge of the tub (or on the shower bench) with his legs spread wide. Get down on your knees directly in front of him, hugging his waist, licking his nipples, and massaging his penis. Lather up all around and underneath his penis. Very gently, lift one knee up underneath his scrotum, and with your foot resting on the bottom of the tub or shower, apply easy pressure as you gyrate your knee just enough to give him a slick massage. This may sound like a difficult balancing act, but it's really not—try it!

Finally, don't forget that there are lots of other fun ways to create tantalizing sexual experiences besides intercourse. Get creative. Here are a few more ideas to inspire your sexual confidence.

- *Baskin-Robbins Sex*: For most men, oral pleasures rank high on their list of desired sexual experiences, both the giving and receiving of it. So if you really want to drive him wild, try a little Baskin Robbins sex. Climb on top of him and grant him a little pink spoonful of this and a little pink spoonful of that—a little taste of nipple for a moment, then a little taste of your clitoris. Then move on to indulge in a little taste of his nipples, and a little taste of his penis. Remember that the topmost inch or two of the penis is the most sensitive part, so treat it like an ice cream cone—lick from the top and make your way down. For a double dip of delight, try giving him a taste of you while you're tasting him—also known as a "69."
- *Pretty Pearl Necklace*: If you've been blessed with sizable breasts, don't hesitate to use them creatively. Apply plenty of lotion or lubricant between your breasts, then invite your husband to mount your chest (don't worry, he'll be supporting his weight on his knees, not on your rib cage). Using your palms, squeeze

your breasts toward the center, enveloping his penis in between as he rocks back and forth. For added pleasure, use an edible lubricant (or simply use excess saliva instead of lotion) so that as he thrusts forward, you can tease the tip of his penis with your tongue.

- *Spectator Sport*: On the occasions when you're simply not in the mood to be an active participant, rather than rejecting him, try spectating instead (which can be equally as erotic and arousing!). Give him carte blanche to masturbate however he'd like while you watch and learn what brings him the most pleasure. Maybe even get out that digital camera to film a quick educational documentary (to be deleted later, of course!). By becoming an astute spectator, you'll have the confidence that you know exactly where and how he likes to be touched the next time you're up for full participation. Also be willing to return the favor sometime, giving him an eyeful of what turns you on most so that he can become a real pro at pleasuring you as well!

The Joy of Discovery

One teenager asked recently, "Doesn't married sex get boring, doing the same thing with the same person over and over?" Sure, things can get stale if we let them, but the sexually confident wife doesn't let that happen for long before she develops new strategies to turn up the heat once again. The fun thing about sex in a lifelong committed marriage is that you're never too old to learn some new tricks that will add joy and delight to your relationship.

The ideas discussed in this chapter are merely a fraction of all the sexual activities and positions we could enjoy as we expand our sexual repertoire far beyond the missionary position. I encourage you to seek out more creative ideas in other books as well. We're amazed at how even after eighteen years of marriage (and an active sex life during the vast majority of that time together), we still occasionally stumble on a new position and realize, *Hey! We've never done it this way before, have we?* Greg says that in those moments, he feels like Christopher Columbus, sailing into unchartered territory. I feel like a kid in a candy store, discovering new delights that are sure to become future favorites as I indulge in them again and again.

And I hope that in the years ahead, you'll discover many unchartered territories and indulge in many delightful flavors of sexual pleasure as well.

11

Maintaining Healthy Boundaries

It was my husband's dream vacation—three weeks of camping throughout Arizona, California, Nevada, and Utah with an extended stay near the Grand Canyon. Walking around the south rim of the canyon, Greg was absolutely awestruck, snapping multitudes of family pictures all along the way.

Of course, looking at these pictures once we got home didn't do the Grand Canyon justice. It's one of those wonders that you have to see up close and personal to fathom how beautiful and awe-inspiring it really is. But I did notice something else as we glanced through our photos, something that revealed more about our *human nature* than about Arizona's nature.

As I looked at the plethora of pictures Greg took that day, I noticed the variety of places where we'd stopped to pose and smile for the camera. Some of those places had guardrails, and some did not. Where a guardrail existed, we naturally pressed ourselves right up against it so that the photographer could capture as much of the canyon in the background as possible. Where a guardrail didn't exist, we stood several feet away from the edge for safety's sake while having our picture taken, and very little of the canyon is visible in the background.

Where a safe boundary existed, we felt the freedom to confidently go right to the edge. Where no boundary existed, fear kept us from fully enjoying the magnificent visual experiences that the canyon had to offer.

A similar dynamic occurs with our sexuality. When no boundaries exist between a husband and wife, fear is often present. We fear our partner might hurt us physically, or wound us emotionally. We worry that he might ask us to do something degrading, embarrassing, or even life-threatening. We don't feel comfortable completely letting loose because trust isn't fully established. How can a woman experience and exude sexual confidence if she is fearful, worrisome, uncomfortable, or untrusting? She can't. And that's why establishing and maintaining safe and healthy boundaries is key to fully enjoying the wonder of your sexuality.

Since I began writing about female sexuality, I've received numerous questions from women on the topic of sexual boundaries. I thought it would be helpful to include many of those questions, as well as my responses, in this chapter. Some of the fears and concerns expressed by other women will sound incredibly familiar to you, as perhaps you've wrestled with the same issue at some point in your marriage. Others may shock or surprise you, or even make you laugh. Some may elicit a response of anger or sadness based on your past experiences.

Regardless of how you are affected by each scenario, I encourage you to approach the topic of sexual boundaries with these three commonsense principles in mind:

1. Sex is intended to be pleasurable to both husband and wife.
2. Sex should never be painful to either partner (physically or emotionally).
3. Sex should foster a sense of trust and intimacy in marriage.

With these three guidelines in mind, let's consider some of the scenarios that women often express concern over. Perhaps you've struggled with whether or not one of these sexual activities feels right to you just in the past 24 hours. If so, hopefully you'll have much greater clarity on the issue within the *next* 24 hours.

In most of these scenarios, I'll refrain from being "prescriptive" and try to remain "descriptive." My goal is to help you discern whether this is something that *you* feel comfortable allowing inside *your* marriage or if you'd be better off maintaining a boundary between your sexual relationship and this activity. Other times, I may sound more prescriptive, warning you of why I believe it would be a bad decision to engage in such behavior. Why? Because my goal here is 1) to help you establish boundaries that keep you happy and healthy, 2) to build your sexual self-confidence and help you experience the most pleasure possible, and 3) to foster deeper levels of trust and intimacy in your marriage. With that being said, let's begin with a little trip to . . .

Fantasy Island

There seems to be two schools of thought on sexual fantasy. Some say that it's a perfectly normal aspect of human sexuality and should be embraced, enjoyed, and celebrated. Others say that fantasy (especially that which involves someone other than your spouse) is inappropriate, dangerous, and should be avoided. So which is it? Should we embrace sexual fantasies or try to erase them from our minds? That all depends on who you are, on what you base your sexual ethics, and how you feel about this aspect of your sexuality.

Just as beauty is in the eye of the beholder, sexual fantasy can either seem like an incredibly beautiful or extremely ugly part of your life. For example, Elaine e-mailed:

> I married a year ago, and along with sexual intercourse came sexual fantasies about lots of things that I'm not proud of. I love my husband so much, but in order to have an orgasm I feel like I need to start fantasizing about different people. I can't tell my husband. I feel as if I am being unfaithful to him in my mind, and that would crush him. How can I stop doing this?

Just two days later, I received this e-mail from Randy:

> I have sexual fantasies involving my wife that I wish I could open up and talk to her about, and I'd love to hear hers about me as well. I've heard it could really fuel the passion in a marriage to share your fantasies out loud with each other, and I wish we had that kind of communication in our relationship. How can I approach this with my wife without turning her off, grossing her out, or making her think I'm a pervert?

It's often the case that one partner desires to be more open and verbal about sexual fantasies and the other desires to be more private or even wrestles with guilt over them. At some point, you may find it helpful to have a meeting of the minds about the topic of sexual fantasy, discussing what kind of mental boundaries you'd like to maintain both as individuals and as a couple. But how can you be so vulnerable together without turning each other off, as Randy feared?

First, both partners must recognize that we are sexual beings and sex always starts in the mind. Sexual fantasies are part of life, like breathing, eating, and sleeping. We can't get angry with ourselves or our spouse for having sexual fantasies. That would be like getting angry with him or her for being hungry or sleepy. So the first step to opening lines of communication is for you both to acknowledge to each other, "I'm aware that we each have our own sexual fantasies, so let's make sure we're on the same page with how we are going to handle them."

Each person's fantasies are a reflection of a vast number of things, including early childhood experiences, and rebellion against social taboos or family of origin traditions, for example. Therefore, our fantasies can often serve as road maps to our deepest longings, fears, or unresolved issues. When it comes to the nature of your fantasies, don't expect that you and your husband's should be exactly the same. You are likely as different from each other mentally as you are physically. If his fantasies differ greatly from your own, don't panic. The goal is to find common fantasies that you can share with each other without guilt, fear, or inhibition.

For example, let's look at a dozen of the most popular fantasies for both men and women:

- having sex with an existing partner
- giving and receiving oral sex
- having sex with a new partner
- having sex with someone of the same gender
- having sex with more than one person at a time
- doing something forbidden
- romantic or exotic locations
- being dominant, passive, or submissive
- reliving a previous experience
- being found irresistible
- watching others make love
- trying new sexual positions[1]

Perhaps some things on this list shock or disgust you, while others may send a wave of pleasure through your senses just to imagine them. Again, I'm not prescribing these fantasies, but merely describing them. I'm not telling you to fantasize about all of the things on this list, for I believe there is certainly great value in training your brain and restricting your fantasy life to only that which builds genuine intimacy between you and your husband. For example, anything that involves someone other than your spouse could certainly breed distrust and division, and that does not foster intimacy or confidence. That being said, engaging in some of the aforementioned sexual acts solely with each other (such as oral sex on an exotic vacation) could certainly bring the two of you closer together if you're both comfortable with them.

Regarding the fantasies that don't accomplish the goal of fostering intimacy and trust in your marriage relationship, I don't think you need to waste energy beating yourself up over them. But due to the nature of the human mind, I think an honest, frank discussion about sexual fantasies is warranted in a book such as this.

It's important to understand that *most people fantasize about things that they would never actually want to experience in real life.* Human beings naturally think about the forbidden, but that doesn't mean you have to act on it. Most of us have thought about robbing a bank just to have a million dollars, but would never actually do it. Fantasizing about something that you'd never do in real life doesn't change who you are. You do not have to act out your every desire. You can choose to be a faithful wife with conservative values, even if your fantasies occasionally cross the conservative line. Fantasizing about watching others make love doesn't make you a voyeur. Fantasizing about sex with multiple partners doesn't make you an orgy queen. Don't let your sexual fantasies rob you of your sexual confidence as a faithful wife. Maintain rule over your sexual fantasies rather than letting them rule over you. A good rule of thumb is that if the fantasy 1) involves your spouse, 2) can be shared with your spouse, and 3) is approved of by your spouse, it's going to be a good tool in your confidence toolbelt.

Due to the number of e-mails I receive about this particular issue, it certainly warrants mentioning in this book: *Fantasizing about a same-sex partner doesn't make you a lesbian.* In fact, straight women with high sex drives are twenty-seven times more likely to find both sexes attractive (and therefore more likely to fantasize about a same-sex partner) than straight men with high sex drives.[2] In addition, many women say that in the abstract they would like to have a sexual experience with another woman but never actually do so.[3] According to the sex researcher Dr. Alfred Kinsey, most humans have at least a little homosexuality lurking in our minds, but that shouldn't rob you of your sexual confidence as a heterosexual wife. Again, who we really are isn't determined as much by our fantasies as by who we choose to be in our day-to-day lives.

Remember that what we do with our sexual fantasies can be productive or destructive to our marriage. Quite frankly, many sexual fantasies are far better left as fantasies, especially if they are going to inflict physical or emotional pain on either partner or hinder trust and intimacy in the relationship in any way. If you choose to verbalize your fantasies (see sidebar on page 156), be sure to clarify whether you are suggesting that you want to live out this experience or you are just giving your spouse a peek into your private world for no other reason than to build intimacy and create sexual energy.

A great way to test the waters to see how comfortable you and your spouse feel with revealing certain sexual fantasies is to make a game of *Truth or Consequences* out of it. Present three scenarios, one of which is true and two of which are false. In response to each scenario, your partner responds with his thoughts or feelings about that particular fantasy. Here's an example of such a game:

Kim: I'm going to tell you about three fantasies. One may or may not be my fantasy. The other two are made up things that I don't really fantasize about at all. You tell me how you feel about each one.

Todd: Am I supposed to tell you if I'd want to actually do them, or only if it turns me on to think about you thinking of those things?

Kim: I only want to know how you'd feel if I verbalized these fantasies out loud with you while making love. It's not about wanting to act out on them at all. Okay?

Todd: Okay, I'm ready.

Kim: Scene one is that I'm dressed in high heels and black leather, forcing you to go down on me.

Todd: That's a winner. I'd hope you could tell me if that's what you're thinking. I may even want you to act that one out if you're willing.

Kim: Slow down. That may or may not be my real fantasy. Scene two is that you and I are in a bar together and are approached by another couple who are interested in swinging.

Todd: I wouldn't want to even entertain the idea of sharing you with anyone else.

Kim: Scene three is for you to use a vibrator on me, then make love to me.

Todd: That thought puts a smile on my face.

Based on the information she's so cleverly gathered, Kim can discern whether she wants to keep her fantasy to herself, share it openly, or simply reveal an edited version of it so as to light her husband's fire instead of extinguishing it. ●

Let common sense be your guide regarding if, when, and how to discuss personal fantasies. Never try to drag his out of him if he seems unwilling to share. Never insist on sharing things that make him feel uncomfortable with his own sexuality. Never hurl his or your own fantasies in his direction as a way of venting anger or pointing out his sexual shortcomings. Maintain a playful attitude, and remember that the goal of sharing your fantasies is simply to fuel sexual energy. Also keep in mind our three-question filter to determine what kind of sexual energy you're creating: Does the activity 1) provide pleasure to both? 2) avoid physical or emotional pain to either? 3) foster trust and intimacy in the marriage? If so, great. The sexual energy is positive. If not, you may want to rethink your sexual strategy.

Carefully Consider His Point of View

Although my husband is ecstatic that I'm writing a book to encourage women in their pursuit of sexual confidence, he admitted to having some red flags in his own male spirit in response to some things in this chapter—particularly to the concepts of sharing sexual fantasies, talking dirty to each other, and role playing. Although he may not represent all men, his views will most likely be shared by many, so here's his two cents' worth:

> The topic of discussing sexual fantasies can elicit great
> excitement in your husband, but also great fear. I find it

interesting that the sexual fantasies that arouse a woman during the ten minutes she's making love can have absolutely no effect on her the other twenty-three hours and fifty minutes of the day. However, for a man, it's pretty much opposite. We don't need fantasy during the ten minutes that we're looking at our wife's naked body, but we have to battle those kinds of thoughts the rest of every twenty-four-hour period!

I realize that orgasm is 95 percent mental for a woman; therefore it stands to reason that healthy sexual fantasy may be relied on by women to a certain degree, but females are great at "compartmentalizing" sexual fantasy, drawing such thoughts to the forefront of their mind only when they need to get their sexual motor running. Men find it much harder to compartmentalize fantasy. Those thoughts and images may rev our engines even higher in the bedroom when we're with our wives, but they can also follow us into the shower, the car, the office, on business trips, and so on. This can make resisting sexual temptation very difficult for some men, especially since pornography is so readily available in our society. This is probably true for some women as well.

Throwing caution to the wind and chatting casually about any and every sexual fantasy that comes to your mind can be like feeding a baby alligator. The appetite grows bigger and bigger, along with the power to consume more and more of what it is hungry for, which is usually whatever you've been feeding him all along. So before you fill your husband's mind with what's really going on in yours during the act of making love, take into consideration how differently a man's brain is going to handle all of that information and how vulnerable he can be to temptations outside your marriage bed. Although sexual fantasies are a normal part of every human being's life, know where your personal boundary lines should be drawn, as well as the boundary lines of your husband. Playing inside those boundaries is vital if both spouses are to feel comfortable with the sexual relationship they share.

I agree with Greg wholeheartedly that you also need to take your husband's feelings into consideration about all matters in this chapter, especially if he has reservations. A huge part of sexual confidence includes sexual sensitivity toward your partner and what he finds acceptable and enjoyable. What sounds like "genuine sexual intimacy" to you may sound like nothing more than "overwhelming sexual temptation" to him, or vice versa. He may say things to you in the heat of the moment that either repulse you or awaken unhealthy desires in you that you've tried really hard to put to sleep. Also, our spiritual beliefs often determine our sexual ethics in marriage, so I encourage you to carefully consider what you both feel comfortable with. Pushing for higher sexual intensity at the expense of sexual integrity is far more destructive than productive in any relationship.

Communication is key. Our rule of thumb is that if one of us feels uncomfortable with any sexual activity (even if the activity is just verbal), the other spouse will respect that reservation completely and find satisfaction in those things which satisfy us *both*.

Verbalizing sexual fantasies leads us to another sensitive topic—our sexual vocabulary.

Talk Dirty to Me, Baby! Or Not!

Words have the power to elicit a wide range of positive emotions such as sexual interest, peaceful contentment, and high self-esteem. Words also have the power to elicit a wide range of negative emotions such as fear, shame, anger, and disgust. Unfortunately, words spoken by one person for the benefit of another are often received in a completely different spirit. Just like we mentioned earlier about beauty being in the eye of the beholder, good feelings are found not in the words spoken but in the ear of the hearer.

For that reason, it's imperative that husbands and wives talk about what kind of sexual vocabulary they are most comfortable with. Sharing a common language that builds sexual energy, trust, and intimacy is vital to positive communication experiences. For example, Melinda says, "I often find the words my husband speaks to me in our bedroom offensive. Although he communicates very respectfully outside the bedroom, inside he talks to me like I'm some whore. Do I have a right to speak up about how this bothers me?"

Of course Melinda has that right, and she should exercise it so that her husband can be more sensitive to her needs and desires. Chances are, he doesn't view her as a whore at all but just assumes that such words are acceptable or arousing to her. In fact, they are acceptable to many women, such as Diedra. She says, "I know my husband is a doctor who's accustomed to using proper medical terms with his patients, but I'm not his patient. I'm his wife. Is it really necessary to be so proper in the bedroom? When he says, 'I've wanted to penetrate your vagina all day!' I act interested, but inside I want to laugh and ask if he really thinks he's turning me on with that kind of talk. Should I just go along, or tell him what I really want to hear?"

To answer Diedra's question, let's put the shoe on the other foot. Let's suppose you were saying words to your husband in the heat of the moment that you thought would arouse him but in fact are a turn-off. Would you want to know? Would you want him to teach you what he likes? Of course you would. My guess is that your husband would appreciate the same intimacy.

Just as with fantasy, you can make a fun game out of this. Together, make a list of every sexual term you can think of, both proper medical terms and slang terms. Make two columns, one for your responses and one for his responses. Line by line, read the word and indicate with either a minus sign or a plus sign whether that word is one you'd enjoy hearing in the throes of passion.

Compare your answers, and see what you can learn about each other. Tina's husband learned that she is incredibly turned off by the word "pussy" because she finds it degrading. However, "bush" is a term she doesn't mind, and actually prefers it over "vagina." Jarrod was relieved to have the opportunity to tell his wife, Rebecca, that the word "f– –k" was disturbing to him after watching *Braveheart* (according to the movie, the term originated as an acronym for "Fornication Under Consent of the King," meaning the legal right to rape an Irish girl to impregnate her with English blood). "That's not at all what I desire to do to my wife. I love her. I cherish her. I want to 'make love' to her." So "making love" is Jarrod and Rebecca's agreed-upon sexual term of endearment and arousal.

In addition to choosing words that arouse and inspire, a couple may desire to use words that are more indicative of a script rather than a real-life conversation.

Star of the Show

One of the ways that couples may try stirring things up in the bedroom is by role-playing, creating scenarios with fictitious characters or situations. Some of the more popular role plays are 1) the patient and the naughty nurse, 2) the police officer and the seductive law-breaker, and 3) the staunch professor and the flirtatious schoolgirl.

A woman may feel that pretending to be someone else takes away from the intimacy they experience as husband and wife. This woman will be more sexually confident living in the here and now and pretending to be no one other than herself. That doesn't mean she can't put on her own kind of show to keep things interesting. A sexually confident wife can certainly be sexy enough without adopting a false persona. However, another woman may feel that adding a playful repertoire or two (or ten) to their normal sexual routine creates new passion and energy. She will be more sexually confident allowing her artistic or theatrical side to shine through with her lover. In my opinion, there's no right or wrong here. Find out what your husband finds most exciting, discuss what excites you most, and do whatever makes you both feel comfortable and intimately connected to each other.

One aspect of role-playing, however, deserves some guidelines to ensure that it remains a pleasant rather than a painful experience. I'm not necessarily recommending it (so don't send me any hate mail), but you and your husband may agree that a little S&M (sadism and masochism) role-play might be entertaining. Typically this involves one partner pretending to control the other using mock brute force, and the other partner pretending to enjoy it. One example is the "male professor" using a cushioned paddle to spank the bare bottom of his "rowdy female student," a punishment that only elicits more misbehavior because of her personal enjoyment. S&M can also include bondage, having one person bound by handcuffs, ropes, or ties. This places one person in a dominant role and the other in a submissive role. The submissive person may experience a newfound freedom to enjoy things that they may normally find embarrassing or awkward, and the dominant person may discover a new level of courage in suggesting things that they may be afraid to otherwise.

If this type of role-play appeals to you, be sure to have a code word. A code word is a way of communicating, "Okay, I've had enough," or "This is more pain than I prefer to experience." Pick a word such as "halt" or "red light" and let that be the signal that the game is over, or at least needs to be amended to keep things pleasurably playful. Otherwise, genuine physical or emotional pain can be experienced, and that's never an intimacy booster. Inflicting harm on our sexual partner can be one of the most damaging things you can do to your marriage relationship, so if you're going to play, remember to play it safe and play soft. And make sure you're both comfortable with whatever kind of role-playing game you choose. If not, abandon it and find another way to have fun that suits you both.

Sometimes privately playing out sexual fantasies between the two of you may not seem like it's enough of a thrill. Looking at *other people* can seem a lot more appealing, so let's talk about . . .

Silver Screens and Magazines

Every second of the day, almost 30,000 people are viewing Internet pornography. Every thirty-nine minutes, a new pornographic video is being created in the United States. The pornography industry creates more revenue than Microsoft, Google, Amazon, eBay, Yahoo!, Apple, Netflix, and Earthlink combined.[4] It's a big business, but it can mean big trouble in a marriage when a husband and wife do not agree on whether or not pornography is within their preferred sexual boundaries.

Don't make the assumption that it's always the man who peeps at porn while the women roll their eyes in disgust. It's often the other way around, with one out of three visitors to adult websites being of the female persuasion, and 17 percent of women admitting to being addicted to pornography.[5] In fact, I came into my marriage in 1990 as a woman addicted to porn. My thinking was, *My husband's going to love this about me! I'm so open, so willing, so game for anything!* I was wrong. Greg didn't appreciate the videos I brought into our home. In fact, he asked me to trash them. "I spent years beating myself up for looking at pornography, and I'm finally free from that stuff! Don't make me go back down that road again," Greg explained. "I want to respect myself, and I want to respect you. And I'd never want our children to lose respect for us when they find those videos on our closet shelf!" I was stunned. I had never thought of it that way, but to me personally, it made sense. I had to honor my husband's wishes, and I found that by getting rid of my private porn stash, I became much more focused on my husband during sexual moments. This was by far one of the best intimacy builders for our relationship.

Perhaps both of you feel perfectly okay about viewing pornography together. If so, my intention isn't to guilt you into feeling any differently, although I do want to challenge you to consider how your relationship might grow much deeper without it.

I also want to encourage you to be empowered if you feel negatively about your husband's use of pornography. Be a sexually confident wife, draw the line, and say, "Hey, let's not go there." If he continues to go there without you, feel the freedom to say, "I don't want you going there by yourself, either." You even have the right as his wife to forbid it if it's a hindrance to your marriage and your sexual relationship.

Sometimes this tactic works, as was the case with Greg and me. Sometimes it doesn't. If his continued addiction causes you to feel degraded and devalued, it's cause enough for professional counseling, and there are plenty of treatment centers and accountability ministries that deal with such addictions. *Every Man's Battle* (for husbands) and *Every Heart Restored* (for wives) are two books that can help you work through this issue if needed, and *Every Woman's Battle* can help if you're the one addicted to porn.

Why is looking at pornography any different than engaging in sexual fantasy, role-play, and some of the other things we've talked about? Those other things have involved the two of you interacting *together* sexually. With a visual image of another human being introduced into the mix, the temptation can be overwhelming to disconnect from each other and focus on a completely different person—a person with whom you can never have a sexual relationship, or any other type of relationship for that matter. In fact, most spouses who view porn do so secretly, apart from their mate. And chances are, they're not taking that sexual energy to bed with their spouse. They're taking it into their own hands, relieving themselves of their sexual tension through masturbation, and robbing their partner of an intimate sexual experience in the process. When this happens, sexual energies are squandered in some stranger's direction rather than focused on their spouse. In my opinion, the power of sexual intimacy in your marriage gets completely diluted in the process.

The difference between relying on pornography for sexual highs and looking to your spouse for sexual highs is like the difference between a lightbulb and a laser beam. A lightbulb's rays fan out in a million different directions, which dilutes its power. One lightbulb will barely illuminate one corner of a room. When we're looking at hundreds or even thousands of different pornographic actors, we're spreading our sexual energies in a multitude of directions just like that lightbulb, so it doesn't make for a real powerful experience. There's no special connection with any of the people involved. Eventually, we no longer associate sexual passion with personal connection. Rather, we disconnect. We can easily lose our sexual confidence that just two married people are enough to create a sexual high without the use of silver screens or magazines as a crutch.

However, when we're looking exclusively to our spouse for sexual fulfillment, it's like a laser beam. A laser beam's light rays are all focused in one direction. As a result, it is so powerful you can cut metal or perform surgery with it. By directing our sexual energies toward our spouse, we're able to form a focused, concentrated, powerful bond that can last a lifetime. I encourage you to form that kind of exclusive bond with your husband and to expect that kind of exclusive bond from him as well.

In addition to watching others engage in sexual acts through the use of pornography, sometimes the desire to be watched ourselves can create issues. On occasion, one might experience an overwhelming desire to have an audience, so let's talk about . . .

PDA (Public Displays of Affection)

Onika writes:

> My husband has a thing for making out or even going all the way in relatively public places. We've had sex in our fenced-in backyard (the neighbors could have easily peeked over the fence), in a coed family bathroom at a subway station, and in the back of our SUV in a friend's driveway (we have tinted windows). He says his wildest fantasy and goal in life is to become members of the Mile-High Club, having sex in an airplane. I personally prefer the privacy of our own bedroom, but I'm not sure I want to deny him these thrills if they mean

that much to him. Why is this such a turn-on, and what do you suggest I do?

I can't answer for Onika's husband, but I can say that some people (both men and women) find that such activities create an exhilarating sense of danger. In a recent study, 22 percent of Americans had done it in public within the past twelve months.[6]

While it can be fun to cop a feel under a blanket on a subway ride, public sex is a gamble. If you don't get caught, you walk away a winner. However, if you lose, there may not be words in the English language to describe your embarrassment or the embarrassment felt by the person who discovered your little game. And there may not be enough words to convince the police officer not to ticket you or even arrest you for indecent exposure. In fact, all states have laws against public indecency and nudity. You can be charged with a misdemeanor, resulting in a one-year jail sentence. Sorry, but I can't imagine any orgasm that's worth twelve months behind bars.

So how do you know when to go for it and when to draw the line? Consider best-case and worst-case scenarios. Sexually speaking, best-case scenario is that you experience such an enormous amount of adrenaline coursing through your veins that you fuel a mind-blowing orgasm and create a memory that lasts a lifetime. Worst-case scenario is that you are so distracted by the fear of getting caught that you can't reach orgasm at all and both you and your partner walk away disappointed. Socially and legally speaking, best-case scenario is that you get away with it. Worst-case scenario is that you're discovered by an innocent passerby, reported to the authorities, and possibly face a penalty that proves to be far stiffer than his erection ever was, not to mention the awkwardness felt by friends, family, and coworkers when they have to visit you in jail.

Count the costs and consider whether the odds are in your favor enough to warrant the risk. For example, I mentioned in a previous chapter that my husband and I had sex on our trampoline one evening. We live in the middle of nowhere. If for some strange reason someone had driven up, we'd have been able to hide in the woods until that person left. Even if someone had searched us out and stumbled upon us, we were engaged in private acts on our own private land, and the embarrassment would have been more the visitor's than ours. But if my husband wanted me to do it in a more public place where we could have been fined or arrested (thus jeopardizing our careers and reputations), I'd suggest a cold shower until we can take a steamy one together in our own private bathroom.

I'd also suggest a cold shower to anyone who wanted to act out sexually with someone other than his or her own spouse, which leads us to address the topic of threesomes, swinging, and orgies.

Two's Company, Three's a Crowd

Remember back to our list of the most common sexual fantasies? Having sex with a new partner, having sex with someone of the same gender, having sex with more than one person at a time, watching others make love. Although it's a common fantasy, is it wise to open our bedroom doors to anyone besides our spouse?

Let's go back to our three guidelines discussed earlier in this chapter. First, sex is intended to be pleasurable to both partners. Could a threesome, foursome, or moresome provide pleasure to both partners? Perhaps. But it could also cause enormous pain to you and/or your partner, both physically and emotionally, which flies in the face of guideline number two.

The risk of sexually transmitted diseases or unplanned pregnancy should be enough to inspire you to exclude this from your sexual repertoire. What if your husband accidentally impregnated your extramarital partner? Or unknowingly gave you a disease that another woman gave him? But even if there were no physical consequences, involving other people in your sex life can elicit enormous jealousy and fear of public disclosure. What if she has a better body than you, or your husband seems to prefer her? What if the "other man" falls in love with you and asks you to leave your husband for him? What if he or she brags to someone you know about their sexual escapades involving you? What if they secretly videotape the tryst and attempt to blackmail you, threatening to expose you publicly if you don't fulfill their demands? These may seem extreme, but the cons certainly outweigh the pros, don't they?

Finally, the third guideline (fostering a sense of trust and intimacy) seems impossible in the context of a relationship involving more than two people. For all of these reasons, this is one of those scenarios for which I step out of descriptive mode and into prescriptive mode: *Don't go there.* As I mentioned before, some fantasies are better left as fantasies, and my bet is that this is definitely one of them.

"Threeways are so physically and emotionally exhausting because they do not occur in nature. You never see a gazelle threeway on a [*National Geographic*] special. Because they know better. Only man is fool enough to spit in the eye of God . . . God does not like threeways."

—Lisa Carver, writer

Be Who You Are

While the goal of this book is for women to become less inhibited and more confident in the bedroom, there are certain boundaries that should and must be maintained. These personal boundaries allow you to feel completely safe and secure, which are vital elements in sexual confidence.

Granted, sometimes sexual confidence is best exuded by wholeheartedly saying yes to certain activities that provide pleasure, build trust, and foster intimacy. Other times, sexual confidence is exuded when you feel the freedom to say no to those things that you believe would undermine your sexual integrity and your relational goals. So remember, a sexually confident wife doesn't just throw caution to the wind and say yes to anything and everything. Don't sell your soul just to please someone else, girlfriend—not even your husband!

You have every right to maintain sexual boundaries and to be who you truly feel comfortable being in the bedroom. You have a right to expect sexual sensitivity from your husband. You have the right to demand exclusivity in your sexual relationship. And by exercising these rights with conviction and without apology, your sexual confidence will shine.

Part 5

Overcoming Obstacles

12

Redefining "Normal"

While I was working on my master's degree in counseling and human relations, we were given a series of indepth tests designed to reveal every aspect, nuance, nook, and cranny of our personalities. One such test was the MMPI (Minnesota Multiphasic Personality Inventory), in which almost six hundred questions had to be responded to with only yes or no answers. The test proctor declared, "At no point during this test are you allowed to ask any questions of me or anyone else. If you need clarification about a particular question, you must simply use your best judgment and interpret it as best you can." Clear enough.

However, several minutes into the test, one young man raised his hand and blurted out, "Sir, this question asks, 'Do you have any kinky sex practices?' Can you define 'kinky' for me?"

Honestly, we tried to contain our laughter. The professor, obviously horrified that this student was so blatantly breaking the rules, stood there in silence, refusing to respond. However, one elderly woman in the front row couldn't resist the temptation. She retorted,

"You're *normal* if you use a feather. You're *kinky* if you use the whole bird!" Not even the professor could contain his laughter at that point.

We've probably all wondered at some time in our lives, *Am I normal, or am I kinky? Is my husband normal? Is what we like to do normal?* When it comes to sexual expression, "normal" can be extremely difficult and even detrimental to define. What is normal or pleasurable to one person or couple isn't necessarily normal or pleasurable for another. I agree with Dr. Alex Comfort, sexologist and author of *The Joy of Sex,* when he said, "There is no norm in sex. Norm is the name of a guy who lives in Brooklyn."

Indeed, our sexuality is as unique as our fingerprint. No two people have ever had identical sexual experiences, desires, repulsions, or fantasies. In order for you to overcome any mental obstacles to being a sexually confident wife, let's discuss a few "blue issues" and "pink things" commonly presented.

Blue Issue #1: *Is it normal that my husband wants sex practically all the time?*

While not all men want sex all the time, most crave it quite often. For some guys, "often" means a few times per week. For some, it can mean every day, or even multiple times per day on occasion. And if he isn't asking for it, he may still be thinking about it. Many men report thinking about sex dozens of times per day, and that's just before lunchtime. This doesn't make him an animal but merely a healthy, high-functioning sexual male.

Why is this so hard for some of us to wrap our female brains around? Because we often view sex as something we do when we're horny or aroused (more about the female sex drive when we talk about "pink things" in a moment). But men usually have a much broader view of sex than women. To the male mind, body, and soul, there are the following:

- *boredom sex*—"What better way to bring some excitement into my day?"
- *celebration sex*—"What's happening is so great we should celebrate with great sex!"
- *stress-relieving sex*—"The only way I'm ever going to get my mind off work is to make love to my wife!"
- *post-exercise sex*—"Now that I've had this great workout, I'm ready to chase my wife around the house!"
- *bonding sex*—"I just want to feel the warmth of my woman next to me."
- *comfort sex*—"I'm hurting so badly on the inside that I long for a soothing sexual touch on the outside."

In case you need it spelled out more clearly, men use sex for A-L-L kinds of reasons. This is just how they are wired, and a sexually confident wife's goal will always be to affirm that part of her husband's sexuality rather than make him feel abnormal.

In addition to connecting sex with all sorts of varying emotions, men also are wired physically to desire sex often because they are high testosterone producers. Testosterone is the hormone primarily responsible for our sex drive. Typically, men produce far more testosterone than women, which results in their having bigger muscles, coarser body hair, deeper voices, and sexual organs that often stand at attention for no reason at all. And the more testosterone a man's body produces, the more often he's going to desire sex. Don't chastise him for it. Celebrate the fact that his masculine body functions so fully!

Recently Greg and I attended a convention where we stayed in a really nice hotel room—without kids—and our first day's schedule was incredibly light. Perhaps it was boredom sex he began craving, or celebration sex over being at the convention alone together, or stress-relieving sex because he typically hates conventions. I don't know the reason, but Greg desired sex as often as he craved food that first day. In the early years of our marriage, I would have questioned, "Is this normal?" I might have gotten on my high horse and looked down on him. I may have even thought, *He's just using me as a sexual outlet.* However, as a more mature, sexually confident wife, I was flattered. Rather than turning him down, I let him turn me on, and his high testosterone production fueled passionate playtimes following breakfast, lunch, and dinner!

If you've read this and thought, *Ha! It's more normal for us* never *to want to have sex,* then sit tight. Chapter 14 is for you.

Blue Issue #2: *Is it normal that my husband wants to engage in anal sex?*

In my conversations with women (and their husbands) about this particular topic, it seems as if most people gravitate toward one end of the spectrum or the other. Some say, "Anal sex is dirty, nasty, and gross! It makes my stomach turn to even think about it!" while others say, "Don't knock it until you try it! It's great!" So which is it? Gross or great? That all depends on whom you ask, and both feelings on the matter, even though they are worlds apart, are perfectly normal.

Because anal sex can be such a sensitive topic, let's dive slightly deeper into the issue and talk about the dynamics involved when one partner wants to engage in anal sex and the other partner isn't nearly as game. Who gets their way here? In my opinion, if any sexual act (this one in particular) isn't desired by one partner, the other must submit, surrendering his or her desires out of respect for the other person's feelings. Sex should never hurt—emotionally, physically, mentally, or spiritually. Therefore, if you have any qualms about your husband wanting to introduce a back door guest, you can refuse to open that door. You have that right. It doesn't make you a prude. It just makes you a sexually confident wife—confident about your boundaries and what you do and don't find pleasurable.

However, some women try anal sex out of curiosity and/or a desire to please their husband beyond vaginal or oral stimulation. If you decide to give anal sex a try, experts recommend a good lubricant and a lot of anal foreplay to relax the muscles prior to penetration. Remember, this passageway is accustomed to one-way traffic, so take it slow when introducing anything into the anus. As we mentioned in a previous chapter, it might be good to have a code word so that he knows when enough is enough. Make sure it's understood that you are the one that needs to remain in control at all times during this act. There's a fine line between pleasure and pain when it comes to anal sex. Also know that once his penis is inserted into your anal canal, it should never be inserted into your vaginal canal until after it is properly cleansed.

Of course, to say that a husband is interested in anal sex doesn't necessarily mean that he desires to be the one penetrating. He may prefer to be the one being penetrated. It can be shocking for a woman to discover that her husband enjoys anal stimulation. She may even wonder, *Could this mean he's really gay?* No, men who enjoy anal stimulation aren't necessarily gay. They're just in touch with their pleasure spots, and they aren't afraid to let their wives know about even the most intimate ones. The anus contains thousands of nerve endings (similar to the nipple, the clitoris, or head of the penis), and therefore it's going to provide some rather pleasurable sensations when aroused with your fingers or some sort of object (more about sex toys in the next chapter). Your husband may feel quite comfortable or even eager about having this area aroused. Then again, he may not. Both feelings are very normal, and it's really just a matter of open, honest communication with each other about whether or not anal sex should or shouldn't become an occasional or routine part of your lovemaking.

Blue Issue #3: *Is it normal that my husband completely disconnects after sex?*

The movies paint such a dreamy picture of the intimate moments a couple shares after making love. She snuggles up next to him, and he envelops her with his strong arms. Her dainty head rests peacefully upon his broad, muscular chest. He runs his fingers through her flowing hair and kisses the crown of her head gently. They talk about innermost thoughts and feelings that they perhaps haven't had the courage to discuss up until this magical moment. All of this is what's commonly referred to as "afterglow."

However, our bedrooms aren't movie sets, and basking in the afterglow isn't necessarily hardwired into a man's psyche like it is into a woman's. Most men are more hardwired for a "wham, bam, thank you, ma'am" type of experience. Hopefully he won't use those words exactly, but if his common conclusion to the cataclysmic act of orgasm is to roll over to his side of the bed and begin snoring in seconds, you may be tempted to feel as if you just got screwed rather than made love to. I encourage you not to take his post-sex disconnection personally. Such paranoia can quickly rob you of your sexual confidence. If the afterglow is cut short and he crashes and burns immediately after sex, just smile with the satisfaction that he's invested every ounce of energy he could muster into enjoying your body. There'll be time for afterglow-type moments after he's rested and recovered from your lovemaking frenzy.

Blue Issue #4: *Is it normal that my husband has a sexual fetish?*

I'll never forget how slimed I felt as a young teenager when my boss asked, "Would you like a lifetime supply of panty hose?" I inquired as to what the offer entailed, to which he responded, "I'll give you a new pair for every old pair you give me, but you can't wash them. Give them to me dirty." The overwhelming wave of nausea I experienced in that moment was enough to turn me green and send me running out the door, never to return to that job. While it was completely inappropriate for my boss to make such a suggestion, married partners should actually feel comfortable confiding in their spouse about what really turns them on—even if it's dirty panty hose. In fact, footwear, feet, boots, and shoes top the list of sexual fetishes men admit to. Perhaps it is connected to when he was a little boy sitting safely at his mother's feet and staring up at her womanly body.

A wide variety of other objects can also be a real turn-on for men, such as lingerie, leather, or lipstick. Ponytails can be a real attention-getter as well, perhaps because they project a youthful look, or maybe because of how they expose every subtle curve of a woman's neck. Regardless of what really gets your husband's motor running, if it doesn't offend you, I encourage you to play along. By doing so, you'll enhance not only your own sexual confidence, but his as well.

Take It or Leave It?

People often feel guilty about their sexual fetish because they do not understand its origin or they fear judgment from others. Dr. Thomas Sargent experienced such guilt, then published an article entitled "Fetishism" in the *Journal of Social Work and Human Sexuality*. In the article, Sargent describes himself as a "rubber fetishist and professional therapist, in that order." He relates an incident when he consulted a psychiatrist regarding his love of rubber and the sexual arousal he experienced as a result of contact with the inanimate object. The psychiatrist told him that if he felt guilty, he could either eliminate the guilt or eliminate the rubber. Sargent decided to get rid of the guilt and keep the rubber.[1]

Thinking Pink

Of course, men aren't the only ones who have sexual issues that cause us to wonder, *Is that normal?* Women can be just as quirky in the bedroom, so let's explore a few "pink things" that women may wrestle with.

Pink Thing #1: *Is it normal that I want to have sex all the time?*

It's a complete stereotype to say that it's the man who always wants sex. Many women boldly admit that they possess quite a strong sex drive, even stronger than their husband's at times. Is this normal? Absolutely. And there are several possible explanations. The most obvious explanation is that you may be going through what's commonly referred to as your "sexual peak." Supposedly, men experience their sexual prime in their late teens and early twenties. Women, however, usually experience the most sexual desire in their late thirties and early forties.

There may also be a significant mental, emotional, or spiritual component at work here as well. Perhaps you just have a great understanding of the beauty, appropriateness, and necessity of sexual intimacy in marriage. You value sex. You celebrate your sexuality. You're naturally a sexually confident wife. Hopefully your husband values that in you and celebrates it with you. If not, and you find yourself wanting sex much more often than he does, it can be confusing and bewildering to a woman. Remember that he may not be a naturally high-testosterone-producing person, whereas you may be. Also, he may not have had the same positive messages about sexuality instilled in him. Imagine if the tables were turned and he was far more interested in sex than you. How would you want him to handle the situation? What would be the most effective way he could approach you and encourage you to meet him somewhere in the middle such that you are both fulfilled? Take that same stance with him. Gently, respectfully, and lovingly encourage him to open himself to you so that you can freely enjoy sexual intimacy together without one feeling put upon or taken advantage of by the other.

Again, if you're reading this particular pink thing and thinking, *I can't imagine wanting sex at all, let alone all the time,* then Chapter 14 is for you.

Pink Thing #2: *Is it normal that I prefer to fake it rather than exert the necessary energy to experience orgasm?*

With multiple studies quoting anywhere from 50 to 70 percent of women faking orgasm, I'd have to say this is normal. But just because something is normal doesn't make it healthy. For example, it's normal (commonplace) for Americans to consume massive amounts of junk food during the course of a year, but it's not the best choice. It's a far better choice to grocery shop for nutritious food and prepare it in healthy ways. Yes, it takes more time and energy, but it's a worthy investment. I'd have to say the same about orgasm. It may take longer to experience the real deal versus just faking it and getting it over with. But you rob yourself of ultimate pleasure and sexual confidence by faking it, and you rob your partner of the fulfillment that comes from pleasing your spouse to the point of orgasm. Oh, sure, you can lie to him. You can tell him what you think he wants to hear. But there are no shortcuts to genuine sexual and marital intimacy. I recommend you be honest about your fears, hang-ups, or anything else that may be hindering a true orgasmic experience. Invite him to partner with you to help you overcome this mental obstacle. And if the obstacle is more physical than mental, there's help in the next chapter.

Pink Thing #3: *Is it normal for me to break down and cry or break out in laughter after experiencing orgasm?*

Earlier we talked about how men often collapse in exhaustion after making love, because sex is such an intense physical release for a man. Falling asleep immediately afterward is a common physiological response to physical exhaustion. For a woman, however, sex can create an intense emotional release. And what is the common physiological response to emotional exhaustion? Sometimes it's tears, even though she doesn't know why she's crying. There's nothing particularly wrong. She's not hurting or angry. Yet tears flow freely down her cheeks. These tears are an outward sign of an inward truth—that something has touched her heart in a deep, penetrating way. Consider these tears of passion and celebrate the fact that you are so in touch with your feelings.

Other times, a woman's response to the emotional release that sexual intercourse and orgasm provide is laughter—pure, unadulterated, hysterical laughter. This, too, is perfectly normal, and an outward sign of what's taken place on the inside. Sexual intimacy should elicit great joy, and it's okay to let that show. Just make sure your husband understands that you are laughing *with* him, not *at* him!

Pink Thing #4: *Is it normal that my body makes some strange sounds during sex?*

I find it funny that the only sounds you hear during a sexy lovemaking scene on television or in the movies are a little moaning, groaning, heavy panting, and a flowery musical score in the background. In all my years of lovemaking, I've never heard music while making love unless I turned on the radio before climbing in bed. What I have heard numerous times, however, are some rather graphic sounds—sounds that never make it into the movies! Obviously, Kendra's heard them, too . . .

> My husband and I enjoy making love doggie-style, with me on my hands and knees and him entering from behind. One thing I do not enjoy, however, is the embarrassing sound that comes out of my body afterward, or sometimes even during the act. I don't know of any other way to describe it other than to say it sounds like a big fart, only it's coming out of my vagina instead of my behind. Is this normal? And if it is, why do I feel so humiliated by it?

Actually, this sound is so normal that there's been a slang term coined for it—a "queef." (I was educated about this term by an intelligent group of teenagers on a sexuality retreat I led back in the 1990s.) Basically, a queef is your body's way of expelling air pockets that are forced into your vaginal canal during penetration. And yes, having sex doggie-style seems to make a woman far more prone to creating this unique sound. If you find this embarrassing, you may want to explain to your husband what's really happening so that he'll know it's not flatulence (a.k.a. farting). Learn to laugh about it, as unique sounds (even accidentally farting during lovemaking) are all part of the beautiful dance of sexual intimacy.

"Sex is making a fool of yourself ... That is why sex is so intimate Making mistakes is one of the most revealing and intimate moments of sexual communication."
—*Jerry Rubin, journalist, therapist*

I'll add a random word of caution here. Be sure your husband knows never to intentionally blow air into your vaginal canal to see if he can manufacture the "queef" sound. That can cause an embolism, which can endanger a woman's health.

While we're on the subject of sexual sounds, it's also worth mentioning that some women find it difficult to perform oral sex on their husbands without making a gagging noise, or even throwing up a little bit on occasion because of the gagging reflex. As I'm sure you can imagine, there's nothing that turns a couple off more quickly than the sound of vomiting, even if it's a false alarm! If gagging during oral sex is an issue for you, use your hand (wet with saliva) to massage the bottom half of his penis, and take in only the top half of the shaft into your mouth. This should reduce the depth of oral penetration enough to prevent gagging yet still provide plenty of oral stimulation to the tip of the penis, where it's most pleasurable for him. You can go up and down toward the base with your tongue on occasion (kind of like the way you'd eat an ice cream cone that's melting), but don't feel pressure to take the whole thing into your mouth if it's going to cause a negative reflex action.

Finally, you may not be the only one creating unexpected, not-so-sexy sounds. If your husband accidentally passes gas, don't get bent out of shape. Everyone does it on occasion, and sometimes it simply can't be helped in that particular moment, even if it's a passionate moment. Of course, if he does this on purpose simply because he thinks it's funny, perhaps even fanning the sheets to make sure you get a really good whiff of his flatulence, well, that's another matter—a matter I'll let you take into your own hands.

Developing Mental Confidence

Perhaps there are other "Is this normal?" questions you're curious about. Don't be afraid to consult with a professional counselor or sex therapist if it will give you a greater sense of peace and sexual confidence. However, you might want to save yourself that nickel by remembering that "normal" is nothing more than a thermometer reading at the doctor's office or a setting on your clothes dryer. When it comes to sexual issues, as long as no harm is done and all is kept solely between consenting spouses, just about anything and everything in the bedroom can be considered perfectly normal.

Of course, mental obstacles are just one of the hurdles a woman must jump in order to become a sexually confident wife. There may be other current or future obstacles to overcome as well, so keep reading as we discuss physical challenges and dysfunctions.

13

Rising to the Challenge

was only eighteen years old when I met Joe. I was working as an aide at a nursing home, and Joe was one of my assigned patients that I cared for on the three-to-ten p.m. shift, five days per week. Joe was unlike all of my other patients. He was only thirty-five.

Three years earlier, he and his wife were on a road trip. Joe was sleeping in the backseat while his wife was at the wheel. Feeling sleepy herself, she pulled over to the side of the highway to rest her eyes for a few minutes. She was awakened by a diesel truck plowing into the back of their little sedan at seventy miles per hour. She walked away from the crash with minor cuts and bruises. Joe wasn't so fortunate. He was wheeled away on an ambulance gurney and spent several weeks in ICU. Eventually feeling returned to his body, but because of the brain damage he experienced, complete motor control did not. Later, when doctors concluded there was nothing more they could do, Joe was admitted to the nursing home.

"Where is his wife now?" I asked my supervisor.

"Once Joe left the hospital to come here, she left town," Beatrice explained. "She's never visited him once. She filed for a divorce, and I hear that she's remarried." My heart sank. Every time I took Joe's vital signs or fed him his supper or changed his bedding, I wanted to hug him and say, "I'm so sorry your wife abandoned you just when you needed her most!" The longing in his eyes for human companionship still haunts me to this day.

Three doors down and across the hall resided Alma. Alma was in her late seventies and had been battling skin cancer that had metastasized to some of her internal organs. She had lost her eye to cancer, and much of the skin around her eye socket was black and rough, like a bumpy oil-topped country road. At first I felt sorry for Alma, but that changed within a few short hours when I met her husband, Ralph. He visited her every day, bringing flowers, candy, or a book to read to her. Ralph would often approach me with a sweet smile on his face, slip fifty cents into my pocket, and say, "Here's some Dr. Pepper money for you when you take your break. Thanks for taking such good care of Alma for me." He was crazy about that woman, and he wasn't afraid for anyone to know it. In fact, every few days when he slipped that fifty cents into my pocket, he'd ask, "Do you mind hanging your sign on Alma's door for a little while?"

He was referring to my Do Not Disturb sign. The nurse's aides put the sign on the door to protect the patients' dignity when we were changing their clothes or giving them a sponge bath. I knew Ralph wasn't changing Alma's clothes or giving her a sponge bath. He was being sexually intimate with her. My supervisor had warned me that Ralph would expect that courtesy, and to allow him private time with his wife.

"Some people may think it's sick that an old man would want to have sex with his cancer-riddled wife, but if you think about it, it's really the most beautiful thing in the world," Beatrice explained. I did think about it. In fact, I've thought about it a lot through the years—about what an extraordinary love Ralph and Alma shared, about how much Alma must have needed to know that her husband still found her attractive, even with cancer eating away at her face, about how much of a comfort it must have been for Ralph to escape the loneliness of his empty house to come and enjoy intimate moments with his beloved wife, about how much sexual confidence they both possessed to unapologetically pursue such private pleasures with each other in the not-so-private surroundings of a nursing home. Many times, I've thought, *Oh, I hope Greg and I can love each other like that if we ever face such challenges!*

I've seen other inspiring examples of passionate love and commitment as well, such as Dana and Christopher Reeve's relationship after he was paralyzed in a horseback riding accident. Best known for his role as Superman, Christopher frankly told ABC's *20/20* that the lack of intimacy was the most difficult aspect of his marriage after the accident. However, the couple was able to overcome the obstacles to intimacy. "Let's put it this way—we're not getting divorced," Reeve said. In fact, they continued to sleep in the same bed. "We're as physical with each other as we can be," said Dana, "and we're as close as we can be."[1]

I saw another couple on television one night who conceived a child together *after* the wife was stricken with paralysis from the neck down. I wanted to shout out a big cheer for them as her husband explained, "This child was no accident. Just because my wife has no physical feeling from the neck down doesn't mean we don't still have a passionate, love-filled relationship, or goals and dreams for our family. Just because she can't hold the baby in her arms without help doesn't mean the child isn't going to grow up with a lot of love and all the attention it needs. It requires more effort on my part and the part of our other children, but that's okay. Our family is worth it."

What kind of love do you long to receive? What kind of love do you long to give? The kind Joe had with his wife? I doubt it. Most likely, the kind of love Ralph and Alma, Dana and Christopher Reeve, and this other couple shared is what you aspire to as well. These relationships give us a glimpse into what "in sickness and in health, until death do us part" really means.

Here are a couple more examples of women who've chosen to overcome their physical hurdles and rise to the challenge:

- Beth has struggled with vaginismus since her first gynecological exam as a teenager. This condition causes a woman's pubococcygeus muscle (or PC muscle) to tense suddenly without control, similar to how our eyelids tense when something is coming too close to our eyes. Vaginismus makes any type of vaginal penetration either painful or impossible. But rather than allow this to spoil all her fun, she says, "We've discovered plenty of other ways to pleasure one another and feel close to each other. We refuse to let this ruin our relationship." Way to go, Beth!

- At a women's conference, Julie shared with me in tears about her husband's diabetes, stroke, and resulting weight gain, which pushed him over the four-hundred-pound mark and restricted him to a wheelchair, making frequent showers or baths difficult. These physical challenges left Julie uninterested in oral or vaginal sex, but after a private pep talk about what a vital part sexual intimacy is in any marriage, she took my advice and went home that night and offered her hands for his pleasure. She wrote in an e-mail two days later, "He responded so enthusiastically after feeling neglected for so long. Using the hands God has given us was a wonderful solution. I felt closer to him that I have felt in a long time, and I believe this is only the beginning of the restoration process our marriage so desperately needed." That's the spirit, Julie!

Hopefully you're not facing trials as severe as the ones I've described, but realize that most every marriage will eventually experience some physical challenges or perhaps some sort of sexual dysfunction. The question is "Are you committed to overcoming such physical hurdles when they appear?" If so, let's talk about some of the most common sexual challenges, beginning with those that most every woman must wrestle with every few weeks.

The Monthly Challenge

Sometimes the sexual hurdles holding a couple back are relatively small and minor, yet they can create major havoc in a relationship if we let them. For example, Jacqueline complains that her husband wants to make love even when she has her period. "That just seems so gross to me—so messy and unnecessary. Why can't he just be patient for five days?" Unfortunately, five days can feel like an eternity to a hormonal man, and when you're asking him to give up sex for five straight days every month, well, he might think that's a lot to ask (not to mention the PMS days beforehand when the tension can be so thick that sex is the furthest thing from either of your minds).

If this scenario sounds familiar, I want to challenge you to rethink the situation. You're going to have to deal with your own bloody mess every month regardless of whether you have sex or not, so how does this inconvenience you so terribly? If he's willing to get himself messy, why not let him? He's a big boy. He can clean himself up. If you're worried about staining the sheets, lay an old towel down that can easily be washed come laundry day.

Or perhaps the scenario is the other way around—he doesn't want to have sex while you're menstruating but that seems to be the time of the month that you're the most sexually ravenous. Talk to him rationally and see if you can't come up with a compromise. Suggest that during those days, the two of you could enjoy some good, clean shower sex. Offer to wash him off before he even opens his eyes if it's simply the sight of blood that freaks him out.

If both of you are opposed to sex during menstruation, that's one thing. There's no argument, and since it's not broken, it doesn't need to be fixed. But if one of you wants sex and the other is withholding, it's time for a truce and a new win-win strategy. Ask yourself how far you are willing to bend, and then bend in that direction as often as is necessary to keep the sexual intimacy level high, regardless of what day of the month it is. (Of course, some people refrain from sex during menstruation for religious reasons, which we'll talk about more in the next chapter.)

There is a season of life when a woman doesn't have to worry about her periods at all, yet a new challenge may surface . . .

The Nine-Month Challenge

What joy a couple experiences when they are expecting a child! Not many things in life compare to this level of excitement and anticipation. The downside, however, is that a woman may be tempted to use pregnancy as an excuse not to have sex nearly as often with the father of that child. "You'll hurt the baby," "I'm tired all the time," "I feel too fat to enjoy sex," and on and on the list of excuses can go. If it's unkind to expect a man to go five straight days without sex while his wife is menstruating, it's absolutely cruel to expect him to go months and months until the baby is born—plus a few months more after the baby is born!

Most doctors agree that pregnancy is absolutely no reason not to engage in sexual relations, unless there are extenuating circumstances surrounding a pregnancy that require intercourse to be temporarily off-limits. Talk to your doctor if you have concerns or experience unusual discomfort during sex. If you get the green light on continued sexual relations but just feel uncomfortable (I know from experience that it's sometimes hard making love with a belly full of baby in between the two of you!), try new, more comfortable positions such as scissor sex (discussed on page 145).

If for some reason your doctor says that intercourse is off-limits, that doesn't mean that you can't have some great sexual experiences together. You still need those as a couple, especially before Junior comes into this world and rules your every waking (and sleeping) moment for the next several months! As mentioned in Chapter 10, there are other tantalizing sexual techniques on which you can rely. Nothing says to your husband, "I love you" like a good hand job or blow job when you're out of sexual commission. Or take advantage of what the magical Titty Fairy brings you during pregnancy (significantly increased breast size) and offer a pleasurable pearl necklace to relieve his sexual tension. Just because you're out of sexual commission doesn't mean he is. Also, ask your doctor what sexual activities you *can* enjoy, and you may discover that although intercourse is off-limits, orgasm is not. If that's the case, clitoral stimulation is fair game, and you can enjoy genital massage and oral sex as well.

Remember, intercourse is a small part of lovemaking. Don't lose your sexual confidence (or rob him of his) just because you are expecting a baby.

The Postpartum Challenge

Once pregnancy is a thing of the past, your doctor will tell you how long you should wait before having sexual intercourse. On average, most doctors say that six to twelve weeks is recommended. For those of you who've not experienced this joy yet, your sexual confidence may be threatened by visions of the great black hole. I'm not talking about the one in space, but the one you envision will be between your legs after you pass an eight-to-ten-pound baby through your vaginal canal. I worried about that as well, but my big black hole fears were alleviated the first time I attempted intercourse when my daughter was about ten weeks old. I was actually so tight that post-partum sex was surprisingly difficult.

Every time you breastfeed your baby, the nipple stimulation sends signals to all of your baby-making parts to contract. After several weeks of contractions, your vaginal canal can feel tighter than it did when you were a virgin. But with a little lubricant, finger foreplay, and extreme sensitivity on your husband's part as he's penetrating you, those muscles will soon relax and feel normal once again. The first time you engage in postpartum sex, I recommend that you be on top, or at least in a position where you have more control over the entry rate and rhythm of his penis.

"Recurrent" Challenges

When a woman marries a man, she wants to give him everything— her mind, body, heart, and soul. However, she does *not* want to give him her sexually transmitted disease. Nor does she want to be the recipient of his. Since 80 percent of sexually active adults (four out of every five) will contract an STD in their lifetime,[2] this can pose a challenge.

Jan was honest with James before they married. "You have the right to know in advance that I contracted herpes from a previous partner," she said. "I don't want to pass it on to you, so there may be days when I can play in your playground but you can't play in mine. My doctor says I can have children but may need to have a cesarean section come time for the baby to be delivered. Can you handle all of that?"

Fortunately, James rose to the challenge out of his love for Jan. After twenty-one years of marriage, they have two beautiful daughters but still only one case of herpes. James has managed to remain uninfected because of Jan's caution. She says she can tell when she's about to have a herpes outbreak, and she's been very careful not to throw caution to the wind and get too caught up in the heat of the moment. "I have to think rationally and be practical, which means sacrificing my own pleasure at times for the sake of James's health. Oh, sure, some people say to just use a condom when one partner has a sexually transmitted disease, but a condom would only protect the shaft of his penis, not the base, or his scrotum, or his groin. It's hard enough to occasionally have to deal with the painful herpes blisters myself, so I certainly don't want to risk infecting the man I love."

Speaking of herpes and recurrent sexual challenges, I'm reminded of one we used to face on a regular basis. I'd been married only a short time when I went to my gynecologist asking for an STD screening. Every few months, I'd experience what felt like a painful sore at the opening of my vaginal canal—painful enough to make intercourse or even digital penetration out of the question. With as many premarital partners as I'd had prior to marriage, I was sure it had to be herpes or some sort of sexually transmitted disease.

When the test came back negative for herpes or any other STD that would cause such an issue, I was baffled. My doctor said, "Just come back next time this happens and we'll take a look." I did this three times. All three times my doctor would just examine me and say, "I don't see anything!" Even though she couldn't see anything, I certainly felt something—something incredibly painful. It was a mystery, until I began seeing a different doctor and discussed the issue with him. He suggested it could be a clogged Bartholin's duct. I'd never heard of such a thing. I did some research and discovered that there are tiny ducts at the opening of a woman's vaginal canal that can get clogged on occasion, causing a painful sensation but no outwardly visible signs necessarily. We finally had a diagnosis, but I needed to know the cause.

A few months later, through trial and error, I finally figured it out. I normally purchased unscented maxipads and tampons, but on occasion I'd accidentally pick up a box at the drugstore that contained perfumes or dyes. When I used those, I could guarantee that I'd be out of sexual commission within a few days. The moral of this story is that if you experience a similar recurring challenge, your remedy could be as easy as purchasing unscented sanitary products. A secondary moral is to talk openly with your doctor about the kind of sexual challenges you may be facing. If you don't get satisfactory answers and remedies, feel free to get a second opinion. What baffles one doctor may be a no-brainer to another.

Father Time Challenges

When we were teenagers, the looming presence of our fathers may have kept us from having all the sex we wanted. As aging adults, the looming presence of Father Time may be serving the same purpose.

It's only natural that as our bodies age and begin to function less effectively, our sexual organs follow suit. For a man, this may happen around his fifties, sometimes slightly earlier, sometimes slightly later. Most often, the diagnosis is erectile dysfunction, which basically means he can't maintain a strong erection all the way through ejaculation. It doesn't mean he doesn't love you like he used to, or that he doesn't find you sexy, or that he doesn't enjoy sexual intimacy anymore. It just means the blood flow to his penis isn't as strong as it once was. If obesity is an issue, it could be the culprit, and simply losing weight may heighten his interest once again. There could also be other circulatory issues that need to be addressed, so it's important that he talk to his doctor, since erectile dysfunction can be merely a symptom of a larger health issue. A doctor may suggest a change in diet, some sort of exercises, or some kind of hormonal therapy such as Viagra.

Men aren't the only ones subject to Father Time's effects. As women experience hormonal fluctuations throughout their baby-making, menopausal, and post-menopausal years, their body can experience all sorts of sexual side effects, including an extreme lack of interest. You may think it's no big deal, but it's likely going to become a big deal to your marriage relationship unless he's slowing down at the exact same rate! As the wise old Mrs. Threadgoode (Jessica Tandy) advised Evelyn (Kathy Bates) in the movie *Fried Green Tomatoes,* "You get you some hormones!" Seriously, the solution to your lack of sexual interest could very well be as simple as taking a little pill that your doctor can prescribe, so why wouldn't you explore that option with an open mind? Prescriptions like the new Zestra may be just what the doctor ordered for your lagging sex drive.

Both the male and female body is designed to be sexual. Let your sexual interest be your medical barometer. If that barometer is flatlining, don't hesitate to seek the advice of a medical professional.

Of course, sometimes a couple can experience sexual challenges that have nothing to do with age, or sexually transmitted diseases, or debilitating illness, or monthly inconveniences. Sometimes you just need a little help in the sexual department.

When He Needs a Little Help

There are some couples who have tried multiple times and multiple ways to pleasure each other to the point of climax but find their efforts fall short of the goal. However, all is not lost simply because a couple needs a little help. There are marital aids that can spark a whole new level of interest, arousal, and yes, even climax if you're willing to let go of your inhibitions and give them a try.

Even for younger men yet unaffected by Father Time, maintaining a strong erection to the point of ejaculation can be a challenge for a wide variety of reasons, such as stress, fatigue, and distraction. If that's the case, he may benefit from using an erection ring. An erection ring is basically a circular piece of stretchy material such as silicone that goes over the head of his erect penis and rests snugly at the base. Imagine tying a ribbon at the base of your finger and what this would do to the blood flow to that extremity. Eventually it would turn a pretty shade of periwinkle blue for lack of circulation. Think of the erection ring as that piece of ribbon tied to the base of his penis. It isn't enough pressure to hurt, but it is enough to keep an ample supply of blood trapped in his penis until he reaches an orgasmic state. His wife may not even feel the erection ring, but she will feel the wonderful results of it, especially if it's the kind that has a vibrator at the base for her pleasure as well! Speaking of her pleasure, let's talk about . . .

When She Needs a Little Help

Because a woman can require several minutes of clitoral or vaginal stimulation in order to reach orgasm (sometimes twenty to forty minutes isn't unusual), she may also benefit from a little help from a friend. Some husbands don't mind participating in sexual marathons and have strong fingers, tongues, and erections with which to do so. Others may find it a little tedious or too exhausting to participate in such a marathon very frequently. But with the help of a marital aid, it can be a win-win experience for the couple. Here are a few products you should know about if you're needing a little help in this area:

- *basic vibrators*: Often referred to as personal massagers, most are shaped like a finger or penis, allowing a woman (or her husband) to either rub it against her clitoris or insert it into her vagina. Most are battery powered, but you can find vibrators that plug into a wall outlet and maintain a steady intensity level, which is nice since there's nothing more disappointing in the heat of the moment than a dying vibrator and no fresh batteries around.

- *G-spot stimulators*: There are certain vibrators or vibrator attachments that are specially designed with a curved tip, which provide G-spot stimulation on the anterior side of the vaginal canal when inserted correctly (the tip should be facing the ceiling if you're lying on your back). In order to achieve a G-spot orgasm, the stimulator may need to be moved around slowly using an in-and-out motion. For a refresher course on experiencing G-spot orgasms, refer back to Chapter 8.

- *eggs and bullets*: These small oval-shaped stimulators pack a sexy punch into any lovemaking routine, both for her and for him. They are designed to be used against a woman's clitoris during intercourse, or against her anus, or against the underside of his testicles or anus where he's incredibly sensitive. Some couples find these so arousing to both partners that they own two so they don't have to share!

- *magic fingers*: These are simply latex finger cots that have ribs or nubs on the end, allowing the pad of your husband's finger to become a fabulous "French tickler" against your clitoris. Some are battery-operated, turning his finger into a small vibrator!

- *combination vibrators*: If you enjoy having your husband stimulate your vagina and clitoris at the same time, this is the perfect toy to put in his hands (or into your own hands if he enjoys watching you!).

- *butt plug*: For women who enjoy anal stimulation but fear putting something into her anus that could get lost (any emergency room nurse will testify that it happens more than you'd think), a butt plug with a wide base provides a safer solution. This marital aid allows for "double penetration" with the woman who might desire simultaneous anal and vaginal stimulation. It can also be used for a husband who enjoys anal stimulation, but of course, some things aren't meant to be shared without using extreme sanitary measures. All of these toys I've mentioned should be properly cleaned both before and after each partner's use. There are special sanitary wipes made for this purpose, or you can simply use mild soap and water, being careful to avoid any cords or battery compartments.

Perhaps at this moment everything within you is screaming, "I can't believe she's talking about this stuff!" If the idea of owning a vibrator or marital aid is so offensive to you, then don't own one. I'm not prescribing them for all women but merely describing them for those women who may find these very items to be just the boost they need to add sizzle to their sex life or overcome their physical sexual hurdles. However, I recognize that there may be a few mental obstacles to being the proud owner of a marital aid, so let's look at some of the ideas that may be rolling around in your mind.

- *I don't want my husband to feel threatened by a vibrator.* Before you jump to the conclusion that your husband *would* feel threatened by a vibrator, have you discussed it with him? In my dealings with married couples, marital aids are often welcome friends because they level the playing field and help him overcome his own fears. What fears am I talking about? The fear that his wife will think he's selfish because they only have ten minutes and he wants sex but she requires at least twenty minutes of stimulation to experience an orgasm. So what's a guy to do? Squelch his own desires? Run the risk of offending her by expecting a one-sided encounter? Honestly, some men react very positively to the idea of having a marital aid that can speed up the process or increase her arousal when necessary. In fact, vibrators can send a woman over the edge almost as fast, if not faster, than a man experiences ejaculation. If he can enlist the help of a marital aid when needed or desired, he may feel the freedom to initiate sex much more often, feeling confident that he can pleasure you as fully as he wants to be pleasured himself. Also, it's much more fun for a man to have sex with a woman who is enjoying herself. If a vibrator is all it takes to turn sex from a "marital duty" into a mind-blowing experience for both of you, isn't it worth it?
- *I don't want to get spoiled to the strong sensations of a vibrator and begin to prefer that over intimacy with my husband.* This is an hon-

orable sentiment, and if it's working for you, great! If you're experiencing wonderful orgasms as often as you'd like, and he's not feeling in the least bit overwhelmed by what it takes to get you there, then you probably don't need a vibrator. But if fear that you'd prefer the battery-powered sensations over your husband's touch is the only thing holding you back, let me paint a new picture for you. Why does it have to be either/or? Why can't it be both/and? Why do you feel that you'd abandon one for the other when you could be enjoying both? Keep in mind that ideally (at least in my opinion) vibrators are to be used as a marital aid, not a masturbation aid. If you agree, create a rule that says it's not for individual play but rather to enhance the playtimes you have *together*. Besides, you wouldn't be the only one that enjoys the good vibrations. Marital aids can be just as effective at stimulating men as they are women.

- *I don't want to look at all of the pornographic stuff in catalogs or on websites in order to shop for such products, and I'm certainly not going to walk into a XXX bookstore to buy one in person!* Again, honorable sentiment. I prefer not to look at pornography either, and neither do I care to be seen walking out of an adult toy store with a plain brown paper bag full of who knows what. Sex is personal. It's private. And it's a beautiful means of reinforcing a married couple's healthy relationship. But granted, so much of what you encounter when shopping for marital aids is anything but beautiful or edifying to a married couple. That's why I recommend a company called Covenant Spice (www .covenantspice.com). They carry all the latest and greatest marital aids and intimacy-enhancing products, but you're only shown the products themselves, not a bunch of shocking displays of women getting themselves off, men with erect penises the size of a nuclear missile, or the latest lesbian porn video. It's all good, clean, marriage-building fun at Covenant Spice! They even have a satisfaction guarantee and very discreet shipping, which leads us to the next possible concern.

- *What would the kids think if they found our sex toy?* I can understand a mom's desire to protect her children from such discoveries. But if women can be crafty enough to successfully keep the box of expensive gourmet chocolates safely hidden somewhere in the kitchen, I would think they can be crafty enough to keep a marital toy box locked and safely hidden somewhere in the master bedroom or closet. There are even specially designed cases with combination locks for such a purpose. But even if they are found, is it really wrong for a married woman to own these things? Is it a crime to want the best sex life possible with the man you've committed your life to? Absolutely not. One woman admitted to me recently, "My mother never talked to me about sex, but finding her vibrator in her lingerie drawer was the best nonverbal lesson in sexual freedom I think she could have given me." Indeed, after the shock wears off, realizing that our mothers are also sexual beings can give us complete freedom to embrace our female sexuality as well. We'll talk more about passing the healthy sexuality torch to our daughters (and sons) in Chapter 16.

Before we move on, I want to reiterate that I'm not saying that all couples should own a marital aid. Please don't send me tacky letters and e-mails saying how disgraceful it is that I would even suggest the use of sex toys. Just hear my heart when I say that if you need a marital aid to overcome any sexual challenges, you don't have to apologize to anyone for it. You don't have to fill out a legal form to acquire a permit for one. Neither do you have to approach your priest and schedule a time for confession over the matter. Be a sexually confident woman. If you *need* one, or if you simply *desire* one, don't let society's sexual taboos rob you of your peace of mind in owning one.

Going to the Extremities

In this chapter we've talked about all kinds of sexual challenges, but by no means is our list exhaustive. There are some sexual challenges that can't be overcome—not with a battery-powered toy, or hormonal therapy, or anything else but time and patience. Sometimes it's just not possible to engage in sexual activity, like the time our family spent one month in Honduras sharing one tiny hotel room with our two children, or the time when Greg threw his back out and every position imaginable caused more pain than he could bear, or the time when _____ (you fill in the blank with your own sexual challenge). In those situations, I encourage you to not worry about what's going on or not going on below the belt and focus on the extremities instead.

What extremities am I referring to? You'd be surprised just how bonding it is for a husband and wife to spend time and energy focusing on each other's feet, hands, and head. Greg makes me melt as he rubs lotion all over my feet and hands, and in between every single toe and finger. Whenever I get a manicure or pedicure, I always get compliments on how smooth my hands and feet are, and that's because I have a husband who knows how to show me love in other places besides my crotch. Greg melts whenever I give him a scalp massage, or rub his neck, or kiss his earlobes, eyelids, or the tip of his nose. Hand-to-head, head-to-head, or any kind of skin-to-skin intimacy is incredibly bonding, and much needed whether sexual intercourse is possible or not.

Sexual expression and marital intimacy doesn't always have to be R-rated. When challenges or dysfunctions rain on your sexual parade, life isn't over, and neither does your happy, fulfilling marriage have to come to an end. Find other creative ways to share intimate moments together, and love each other enough to rise above any challenge.

14

Refueling That Lovin' Feeling

One of my favorite movies hit the big screen the year I graduated from high school—*Top Gun.* If you've watched it, you'll most likely recall the famous scene when fighter pilots Maverick and Goose yell, "I feel the need . . . the need for speed!" while doing a big high-five once in the air and again behind their backs. But another scene in that movie touched me on a much deeper level. As Charlie, the beautiful blond flight instructor (played by Kelly McGillis), attempts to give Maverick (Tom Cruise) the cold shoulder in a local bar, Maverick drops to one knee and serenades her with a powerful rendition of "You've Lost That Lovin' Feeling." Cruise's lyrical escapades do the trick, and before long, Charlie is putty in Maverick's hands.

Can you remember a time when you were putty in your husband's hands? I do. I couldn't get enough of Greg's big, strong arms wrapped around me or his soft lips gently caressing mine. I wanted to gaze into his eyes forever and just watch him as he watched my every move, both of us completely mesmerized by the sight of each other. Each time we made love, I melted like a Creamsicle on a hot summer day.

However, as we fast forwarded the tape several years later, we learned that Creamsicles don't always melt. Sometimes they remain frozen, especially when a man's romantic tactics (or lack thereof) don't impress us much anymore. The "putty in his hands" season is a thing of the past, because putty hardens when it isn't kneaded regularly. We lose that loving feeling, or he loses it, or we both lose it. We begin to feel more like roommates than soul mates.

Then what? Does our sex life become just a page in history because one or both spouses lose interest? Some women try to tell themselves that a lack of sexual passion in the marriage isn't necessarily relationship suicide. In fact, many women have admitted (sadly, some out loud to their husbands) that they wish sex didn't have to be part of the marital equation at all. Hello? Could you deal a bigger blow to his ego? Could you cheat yourself any worse than settling for a frigid, celibate lifestyle?

Perhaps you're one of the multitudes of women who've thought that sex is highly overrated. *Au contraire!* I don't think our human minds could ever overestimate the power of a strong sexual connection in marriage. If anything, I think we highly underrate it. But even if we recognize the healthy, emotionally bonding potential of sex, that doesn't necessarily give us an appetite for it. Sometimes we fail to crave that which is healthiest for us. I never crave broccoli or spinach or any other vegetable for that matter. But I find that once I put it on my plate and in my mouth, vegetables aren't so bad after all. In fact, they can be quite good when prepared the right way. The same thing is true of sex. It may not sound all that appetizing initially, but it does satisfy the body and nourish the soul when we surrender ourselves to it. We can learn to enjoy it thoroughly, and even grow to crave it!

But craving sex when we've lost that loving feeling for our husbands can be as unimaginable as craving a big dose of strychnine. Why would women be willing to sign their sexual death certificate just because the passion and emotion dwindle? Because for a woman, that's what sex is all about! If we no longer have emotional feelings for a man, chances are, we no longer have sexual feelings for him, either. That's why refueling that loving feeling is absolutely vital to any marriage relationship that wants to not only survive but thrive.

Of course, women aren't the only ones who occasionally grow cold emotionally and lose sexual interest. Men have feelings, too, and according to many we've heard from over the years, their wives have been stomping on them. "How can I be motivated to have sex at night with the woman who gives me nothing but grief all day?" some men have asked. In fact, one of the most common issues I hear women lamenting over these days is the fact that even though *she's* interested, he's *not*. So let's talk first about how a woman can fan the flames of passion in her own heart, then about how she can fan the flames of passion in her husband's heart.

Fuel for a Woman's Heart

Because women love to talk and get things out on the table, I encourage you to openly and honestly discuss your lack of interest with a trustworthy individual. If you choose to discuss this with your husband, make sure to approach the topic in such a way that he understands your desire to overcome your lack of interest. Choose your words carefully, as again, this news flash can bruise his ego royally. For example, a bad choice of words might be these:

- "I really don't want to have sex with you anymore."
- "I can't stand the thought of being intimate with you."

- "Don't expect me to be sexual. The idea repulses me."
- "Why do you want sex all the time? I never want sex!"

Better choices of words would be these:

- "I love you so much and am very committed to this marriage, so I can't understand what's behind my lack of interest in sex lately."
- "If I seem a little sexually disinterested, please don't take it personally. It's not you, it's me. Do you think I should see a doctor?"
- "Although we've had a great sex life in the past, things seem to be a little difficult for me now for some reason. Perhaps I should see a counselor."
- "I'm feeling emotionally distanced from you these days, and that's troubling me. Is this something we can work on together?"

Why is careful communication so important when a woman has lost that loving feeling toward her husband? Because you don't want to do any further damage by saying things you'll regret later. The wrong words will deflate not just your own sex drive but his as well, and that's simply not fair. If this is your struggle, own it. Invite him to help you, but don't project it onto him.

In addition, we're always quick to assume that it's all *his* fault that *our* emotional boat isn't floating, but remember that men aren't mind readers. They can't instinctively know what it is that we need or desire, especially since a man's relational needs are so different from a woman's. It's our job to respectfully teach him what we need to feel loved and fulfilled in the relationship. We can't *require* that these needs be met, but we can *inspire* it.

For example, there've been many times in the past when I slipped into the deep, dark abyss of "He just doesn't meet my emotional needs," figuring Greg simply didn't love me anymore. I should have softly approached him and said, "I'm missing you a lot lately. Can we spend some time together soon? Maybe go out to dinner and walk around the park?" But no, I was immature enough to believe that he should know what's wrong with me and know exactly how to fix it. I expected him to read my mind. I wanted him to get down on one knee like Maverick, grab my hand, look deeply into my eyes, and wail, "Bring back that lovin' feeling, cause it's gone, gone, gone, whoa-oa-oa!" But guess what? It didn't happen. And when it didn't happen the way I fantasized it should, I got angrier—and lonelier—and I was robbing *myself* of every loving feeling I ever had for him.

Hopefully, these immature escapades are a thing of the past. I've seen glimmers of hope that I've grown up a little since then. A few weeks ago, after several stressful days of not having time to emotionally connect with Greg, I walked up to his side of the bed, looked him in the eye, and just said, "Will you hold me like a baby?" Greg propped himself up on pillows, sat me down in his lap, and cradled me in his arms. His tenderness started my flow of tears onto his chest, and I confessed, "I've been angry with you for not making time for me lately, but I realize I haven't made much time for you either. Will you forgive me?" Humility, warmth, and softness will refuel that loving feeling in your own heart much faster than being prideful, cold, and hard.

Maybe you are thinking, *But I've built such a thick wall of bitterness and resentment toward my husband that I can't imagine asking him to hold me like that!* Perhaps it's time to tear the wall down and turn it into a bridge instead. In fact, I encourage you to make it a point at least once each week (or several times a week is even better) to approach your husband and either ask him to hold you or offer to hold him. Even if you don't feel like it in that moment, as humans we need physical touch, and marriage is the primary relationship where that need should be fulfilled.

Remember that it's easier to act your way into a new way of feeling than to feel your way into a new way of acting. Reach out. Touch him. Take his hand and put it on whatever body part most yearns to be touched, whether that's your cheek, your shoulders, your thighs, your earlobes, or wherever. Offer him your hand and tell him to do the same. Don't underestimate the power of effective communication and tender touch. They are the key to refueling your loving feelings.

If for some reason you don't feel you can confide in your husband about where you are emotionally during this season of your life, enlist the help of a professional counselor or trusted female confidante. Most every woman I know has experienced at least one if not multiple seasons of sexual disinterest in her life. Sometimes it was a hormonal issue. Sometimes it was due to an extended episode of depression. Other times it's because of pent-up hostilities toward her husband, or unresolved wounds from negative childhood experiences such as abuse or incest. Regardless of the reason, don't suffer in silence. You are a sexual woman, with sexual needs and feelings, even if those feelings are temporarily numbed for reasons you don't understand. Let someone help you unlock the mystery behind your sexual paralysis so that you can be healed and whole once again.

If it's your husband's lack of sexual or emotional interest that has you baffled, let's consider what you can do to fan his flame of passion.

Fuel for a Husband's Heart

Over the past eighteen years, Greg and I have enjoyed seasons where we make love often. But there's also been many seasons when there was little or no sex at all. Perhaps Greg really was interested in sex during those times, just not with me. While it's normal for some men not to be in the mood on occasion, it's not normal when the occasion lasts a long, long time. Even the most sexually confident wife can feel devastated by a husband who seems to have lost sexual interest in her. For example:

- Misty e-mails, "I read often of women not wanting to have sex with husbands, but what is a woman to do when her advances toward her husband are not returned? What of the women who want sex and their husbands withhold purposefully? How do you remain sexually confident in an unresponsive situation? This has been an issue at periods of time in my life, and I'm a tall, slender, personable, adventurous young woman with every reason to be confident in what I have to offer."

- Maya confesses she's not a very sexually confident wife because of her husband's lack of interest in her and his extreme interest in other women. She bemoans, "All his affairs have left me wondering what I've been doing wrong. Some of these 'other women' have even said things like, 'If she was woman enough, he would not have had the affair in the first place.' My counselor tells me that a husband's infidelity is never his wife's fault but rather an indication of his own sexual insecurities, but I still can't help but feel like something must be wrong with me."

Maya's counselor is right, and while it may be difficult to understand what's behind a straying husband's sexual misconduct or a faithful husband's lack of interest, let's take a look at some of the possible factors involved. Unresolved childhood issues may be haunting him, just like they often haunt women, affecting his ability to perform. He may be drawn to pornography and masturbation rather than mustering the energy that relationships require. Extreme job stress or financial burdens can drive him to distraction from things that are ultimately most important to him. There may be some medical or hormonal issues putting a crimp in his sexual style.

I don't offer these possible explanations to alarm you, but simply to make you aware of the fact that there's a whole host of reasons why men might lose sexual interest in their wives. However, based on the e-mails we often receive from men, Greg and I believe the most common reason a man loses his sexual appetite for his wife is because she loses respect for him. For example, Albert laments:

> Why is it that women think they can be rude, demanding, and disrespectful to their husbands, then expect that everything should function normally in bed? When my wife rides me all evening about how I don't help out enough in the house or with the kids, or how I don't bring home enough money for her to pay all the bills, or how I don't pay her enough attention or meet her emotional needs, the last thing I want to do is cuddle up next to her and make love.

Think about it. If a man treated a woman harshly during the day, would she be eager to let him touch her that night? Not a chance. This dynamic works both ways. Sometimes a woman expects that her husband's heart and penis should be made of steel, built to withstand the most disappointing and frustrating of relational dynamics. But he's no robot. He's a human being with feelings and emotions, and he needs to be somewhat affirmed in order to feel aroused.

"After fifteen years of marriage, they finally achieved sexual compatibility. They both had a headache."
    —*Anonymous*

Greg and I explore each of these concepts on a much deeper level in our book *Every Woman's Marriage: Igniting the Joy and Passion You Both Desire*, but I want to at least touch on four key concepts here since this is such a common problem in marriage. Before he wants his favorite three-letter word (S-E-X), consider some of his other favorite words:

- His favorite four-letter word: N-I-C-E.
    If your husband has ever felt that you are far nicer to the delivery boy whom you barely know than you are to him, he may lose sexual interest. If your husband sees you being sweet as pie to everyone in your circle of friends but you act more like the Wicked Witch of the West with him after everyone else has gone home, he may lose sexual interest. If you scream at him because of his shortcomings and berate him for not living up to your expectations, you can guarantee that he's going to lose sexual interest. Being nice, not just some of the time but as a general rule, goes a long way. We all have our momentary lapses on occasion, but if you want a sexually interested husband, your "nice" days need to far outweigh your "not-so-nice" days.
- His favorite five-letter word: H-A-P-P-Y.
    Because men feel relatively responsible for their wife's happiness, one of the cruelest things a woman can do to her man is to never be happy. Simply stated, no one likes to be around an

unhappy person, and certainly no one desires to make love to an unhappy person. Sure, there are lots of things that can make us feel unhappy in any given moment. The dog chews up our favorite shoes. The kids won't stop fighting. The car needs a complete transmission overhaul just when we can barely afford the next tank of gas. But lasting happiness, true joy, and genuine contentment is something that women can bring to the surface from deep within themselves, even when things aren't going the way we'd planned. Happiness is a key element in anyone's life, marriage, and sexual relationship, so even when life seems to take a downward spiral, find a reason to rejoice and *choose* happiness.

- His favorite six-letter word: F-R-I-E-N-D.

When you think of a friend, you think of someone who makes you feel good, someone you enjoy spending quality time with, someone you desire to please. Often when we think of friendship, we think of our girlfriends. However, our husband needs to feel as if our friendship with him holds a special place in our heart. This is usually easy during the honeymoon phase, but sometimes we get lax and begin to take our friendship with Hubby for granted. We aren't as intentional about scheduling quality time together, and we overlook opportunities to strengthen our relationship. Don't neglect your friendship with your husband! Bless him with words of encouragement. Be patient with him as he chooses to do things his own way rather than your way. Provide much-needed physical touch through hugs or holding hands. Offer to help him with a project the same way you would for one of your other friends. Rather than taking him for granted, take the time to show your husband that he's still your best friend—a friend with whom you share special sexual privileges that no other friend gets to enjoy!

- His favorite seven-letter word: R-E-S-P-E-C-T.

  While a woman's greatest desire is to feel loved, a man's greatest desire is to feel respected. To respect someone means to esteem him highly or to appreciate who he is as a person. I found out just how deeply entrenched the need for respect is in a man's soul when my son was just ten years old. His fourth-grade teacher gave the class an assignment for which the students had to write what they'd like written about them on their tombstone someday. Matthew declared, "I want my tombstone to say, 'Matthew Thomas Ethridge: A Respected Man of God'."

  Amazed at his boldness and certainty, I inquired, "What about 'Matthew Thomas Ethridge: A *Beloved* Man of God'?" thinking that surely to be *beloved* was a higher compliment than being *respected.*

  However, Matthew obviously didn't agree. He retorted, "No! It has to say 'Respected'!" Out of the mouths of babes flows the unadulterated truth. Men of all ages have a deep-seated need for respect, and my husband says it's something men never outgrow—not in their forties, sixties, or even eighties. No matter how much you love him, if you speak to your husband disrespectfully, you can bet his sexual appetite for you will dwindle. Esteem him highly, and his sexual desire for you will skyrocket.

Although I can't declare that this is always the case, I truly believe that if a woman is consistently being nice, happy, friendly, and respectful toward her husband, there's no way he's going to be disinterested in connecting emotionally and sexually with her. Commit at least thirty days to projecting this attitude toward him, and watch his heart melt like butter toward you.

Of course, even when a man is really trying his best to make his woman feel loved, cherished, and desirable, it often doesn't seem like it's enough. Greg has accused me many times of having a "Grand Canyon of emotional needs" that he could never completely fill. He's right. He can really go all out on a Monday, but if he doesn't keep up that same romantic pace all week, by Friday I'm tempted to cry out, "Don't you love me?" Fortunately, I've become a great deal more secure in our marriage, especially since I learned the difference between . . .

Passionate Love and Companionate Love

Believe it or not, some scientists have become increasingly interested in studying the reasons that so many couples seem to "lose that loving feeling." In fact, the belief is widely held that there is actually a biological explanation for this common phenomenon.

> The high of passionate love doesn't last forever. The body builds up a tolerance to the natural chemicals in the brain associated with being in love; more and more are needed to feel the same level of euphoria. Some people interpret the corresponding decrease in sexual energy to mean they are no longer in love, and indeed for some it does mark the end of a relationship. However, rather than an end to love, it may be a transition into the longer-lasting companionate love.
>
> It appears that the brain cannot tolerate the continually revved-up state of passionate love. As the newness of passion fades, the brain kicks in new chemicals, the endorphins, natural morphine-like substances that calm the mind. The excitement may diminish, but the security of companionate love can provide a different, not necessarily lesser, pleasure.[1]

In other words, losing the "passionate" feelings once the honeymoon is over and the newness wears off the relationship is almost a guarantee. But it *doesn't* mean we have to lose the companionate feelings we have for each other.

Think about it. If we can't allow the relationship to mature into this higher form of companionate love, we may be tempted to go looking for passionate love elsewhere. It's certainly out there to be found. Every new relationship can create that "lover's high," but it will always wear off eventually.

Instead of going from guy to guy every few years looking for someone new to spark that loving feeling in us, let's make life much easier on ourselves and everyone around us. Let's simply refuel the loving feelings we have for the man we've committed our lives to, and learn to appreciate the companionate love we share.

15

Overcoming the "Church Lady" Syndrome

n the fall of 1997, I was speaking to a group of parents about pro-actively instilling sexual values in teenagers. In a sea of faces typi-cally including men and women in their thirties, forties, and early fifties, this one little blue-haired old lady stood out of the crowd. She was sitting perfectly upright in her lavender pantsuit, knees and ankles pressed together, black patent leather handbag resting in her lap with her clenched fists firmly gripping the handles. She sat wide-eyed through the entire ninety-minute presentation, barely moving a muscle except to scratch her blue-haired scalp. I tried not to let the thought distract me, but I couldn't help wondering the entire time, *What in the world is this woman thinking about all of this sex talk?*

After the session was over, the elderly woman, hanging on the arm of her adult daughter, approached me at the front of the room. The daughter introduced herself first, then introduced her elderly mother. As we engaged in conversation, I began bracing myself, assuming that this prim and proper "church lady" was about to lambaste me for talking publicly about S-E-X! I could almost envision her asking, as the comedian Dana Carvey often did on *Saturday Night Live,* "Who possessed you into talking about such a vile thing out loud in church? Hmm, let's see . . . Who could it have been? *SATAN???*"

After exchanging a few pleasantries, the younger woman said, "I just want to thank you for your courage in speaking out about these important issues!" Surprised and relieved, I reached out to give her a hug. As I did, her mother chimed in with her two cents' worth. She said to her daughter in a slow, sweet Southern drawl, "Honey, you are so lucky to be living in a day and age where we can talk about this! Why, I could never even tell your father that I *liked* what he was doing to me at night!"

I've never been so tempted to burst out in laughter and cry tears of relief at the same time! I thought, *Thank God for people who get it!*

Of course, I haven't always been so lucky when I speak to adults. I've had a handful of real, live "church ladies" respond very differently to some of my presentations. One woman insisted, "This is shameful! There's so much sex in the world already, and now we have to bring it into the church?" Another said, "This is a holy place of worship! You're going to talk about SEX *here?*"

If these women find talking about sex in church so disturbing, are they really able to indulge in it freely in their bedrooms? I'm guessing not. It's as if they believe God created our heads, shoulders, knees, and toes, but that our genitals were all the devil's doing. Over the past twelve years of speaking about sexuality in a spiritual context, I've found it painfully obvious that in some women's minds, talking about sex in church is as taboo as marching into a Weight Watchers meeting with a grocery cart full of Häagen-Dazs!

Speaking of ice cream, my favorite is chocolate and vanilla swirled together, which brings to mind the perfect illustration of how I feel about the "church lady" syndrome.

The Power of Swirling Two Great Things Together

One of my favorite places to dine is a casual restaurant called Jason's Deli. The real reason I go there isn't the yummy soup, fresh salad, or delectable sandwiches. The real reason, I confess, is the free soft-serve ice cream. To me, nothing tastes better after a light lunch than a cool and creamy chocolate and vanilla swirl cone!

My husband, on the other hand, well, let's just say he's a "plain vanilla" kind of guy when it comes to his ice cream. He's probably the only person on the planet that walks into a Baskin-Robbins, peruses all thirty-one flavors, and still orders vanilla every time. My kids and I get a big kick out of this.

But once I convinced Greg to let loose and take a walk on the wild side. I presented him with a small dish of chocolate and vanilla swirl, insisting he give it a try, if only to entertain us for a moment. We all anticipated Greg's response as he dipped his plastic spoon into the mixture, brought it to his lips, and shoved it into his mouth. After a split second of mental consultation with his palate, he declared, "Ugh! I don't like chocolate ice cream! Just give me my dear old vanilla and I'll be a happy man!"

That's basically what those "church ladies" were saying, too. "I like my spirituality all by itself! Don't try to mix any sexuality in with my theology!"

Me, on the other hand, I like vanilla okay, and I like chocolate okay, but you swirl those two together and WOW! My taste buds sing! I believe the same is true with sexuality and spirituality. Each is great, but when you experience them together, that makes both of them all the more satisfying.

For that reason, I don't feel this book would be complete without considering the role that spirituality can play in our sex lives—both for the positive and for the negative.

A Spiritual Wet Blanket?

I recently decided to conduct a simple, random survey of my own about how spirituality might affect a person's view of sexuality, and vice versa. I approached several local college students (some married and some single) and asked each one, "Do you believe there is a God?" If they answered positively, I followed up with the question "How do you think God feels about sex?" The results may (or may not) surprise you:

- "Uhhh . . . He doesn't like it?"
- "Well, He doesn't do it, that's for sure!"
- "He abhors sex because it's a sin!"
- "He tells us we shouldn't do it!"

With an entirely different group of students, I approached my line of questioning in the opposite order. "How do you feel about sex?" I asked, then followed with the question, "Do you believe there is a God?" In answer to the first question, I'd usually get responses such as "I love sex!" or "Sex is awesome!" But when I gently sprang the second question on them about God's existence, it was as if they'd been confronted by a *60 Minutes* camera crew. Some ducked their head, lowered their eyes, or lifted their shoulders as if they were trying to make their head disappear like a turtle in a shell. They obviously felt like a child who'd just been caught stealing from the cookie jar before dinnertime.

Granted, my personal poll is a far cry from the most scientific study in the world, but it confirmed my suspicion: When we look at sexuality through the lens of spirituality, *many view sex in a negative light.* If we look at spirituality through the lens of sexuality, *many view God in a negative light.* Why is that?

Some of us were raised in religious homes where spiritual disciplines such as prayer, personal study, and worship attendance were practiced but nothing was ever taught about sexuality. A "don't ask, don't tell" rule silently loomed large over many family living rooms. We never learned to view sexuality through the lens of spirituality at all. We assumed sex to be something altogether inappropriate, or else we'd be talking about it in our homes, in our Sunday school classes, and in our churches, temples, or synagogues.

What happens to a woman when she grows up with the mentality that sex is bad and God doesn't approve of it? She feels as if she can't have both. She must choose. God, or sex. Vanilla, or chocolate. But not both. You can never have both. Married women sometimes falsely assume that if they freely engage in a sexual relationship with their husband, they'll be "bad girls." After all, the one thing most religious homes did instill in their daughters is that "good girls don't."

But I've got great, life-transforming, earth-shaking, marriage-altering news for you, girlfriend. You *can* have both. You can enjoy spirituality *and* sexuality all swirled together—with whipped cream, rainbow sprinkles, and a cherry on top!

Tommy Nelson, pastor of Denton Bible Church in Denton, Texas, and creator of the *Song of Solomon* video series on love, sex, marriage, and romance, says that mankind has a tendency to think that anything enjoyable must be bad for us. As a result, the church often has a pattern of "throwing out the baby, the bath water, and the rubber ducky" when it comes to pleasurable things like music, films—and sex.[1]

A Case for Combining the Two

Regardless of what your religious beliefs may be, as a married woman you can indulge freely in both sexuality and spirituality. In fact, they're much better combined!

As I began brainstorming for this book, I made long lists of the numerous obstacles and hurdles that hold women back in the bedroom. Some were mental obstacles, some were physical obstacles, and some were emotional obstacles. But as we discussed in Chapter 2, our sexuality is comprised of four unique components—the physical, mental, emotional, and spiritual—and with the spiritual component being the deepest one of all, I knew there was no way I could write a book about becoming a sexually confident wife without tackling some of those deep-seated spiritual obstacles that can so easily take the wind right out of a woman's sexual sails. So I began questioning, "Is there any major religion in which sex between a husband and a wife is forbidden, or even discouraged?"

After lots of research, I want to declare with confidence, *No! There isn't!* Buddhists celebrate married sex. Christians celebrate married sex. Jews celebrate married sex. Muslims celebrate married sex. If any religion openly discouraged sex within marriage, the entire population would have died off within a generation or two! So why shouldn't we swirl spirituality and sexuality together and enjoy both?

I believe the best-selling author (and husband) Philip Yancey would agree. In *Designer Sex,* he writes:

> In one sense, we are never more Godlike than in the act of sex. We make ourselves vulnerable. We risk. We give and receive in a simultaneous act. We feel a primordial delight, entering into

the other in communion. Quite literally we make one flesh out of two different persons, experiencing for a brief time a unity like no other. Two independent beings open their inmost selves and experience not a loss but a gain.[2]

In other words, spirituality and sexuality swirled together gives us even greater insight into both pleasures. Not only can God teach us how to have a healthier sexual relationship in marriage, but our sex life can also teach us how to have a healthier relationship with God.

For those of us who grew up in religious homes, all of the "good girls don't have sex" messages were intended to derail us not from sex but from sexual immorality (or sex outside of marriage), which most religions do oppose. However, sex *inside* of marriage is an entirely different matter. And all major religions endorse healthy sexual expression in marriage not only for the purpose of procreation but also for the purpose of mutual pleasure, intimate companionship, and marital unity.

> "It was never dirty to me. After all, God gave us the equipment and opportunity. There's that old saying, 'If God had meant us to fly, he'd have given us wings.' Well, look what he did give us."
>
> —*Dolly Parton, singer, songwriter*

Too bad Sophie has failed to fully grasp these concepts. She says,

> Although I am more open to sex as a married woman than ever before, there is still a part of me that wants to squash any ideas of doing anything sexual beyond basic intercourse on occasion. I guess I fear actually enjoying it, or being judged if I really let

loose and unleash my sexual desires. It just seems easier and safer to limit myself sexually and not have to deal with the fear or guilt.

If Sophie's sentiments ring true with you, let me ask you this question: *Who would judge you?* Who can condemn a married woman for not just "fulfilling her marital duty" but actually enjoying it in the process? Anyone would be unfair to pass such a judgment. Husbands long for their wives to enjoy their sexual relationship, and so does God. Isn't that what He designed our bodies to do, especially when you consider that the clitoris serves absolutely no other biological purpose than to provide a woman pleasure? I believe one of God's greatest desires is for His children to get comfortable with their sexuality so we can freely enjoy the gift He's designed for us.

A Perfect Gift from a Perfect God

Imagine this scenario. I know my daughter absolutely loves sushi. So to show her how much I love her, I make an entire tray of the most exquisite California rolls you've ever seen or tasted. I leave them on the top shelf of the fridge with a note that says, "Enjoy! I love you!"

But days later, I notice she hasn't touched them. I inquire, "Erin, why have you not enjoyed the sushi I made for you?"

She replies, "I was afraid you'd judge me if I enjoyed them too much."

I respond, "What? But I made them especially for you—for your pleasure! Why in the world would you fear I'd judge you for indulging in them?" If anything, I feel hurt that she hasn't allowed herself to enjoy them at all.

Doesn't make sense, does it? Nor does it make sense for us to fear indulging in sexual intimacy within marriage when this is the exact exquisite gift God has created especially for our enjoyment. Perhaps rather than fear offending God with our sexual expression, we should fear offending God by our lack of it.

Granted, there are some religions that expect followers to abide by certain sexual guidelines, such as abstaining from sex at certain times during a woman's menstrual cycle, or refraining from using artificial forms of birth control. I encourage you to talk openly with your pastor, priest, rabbi, or spiritual leader about any spiritual obstacles you are facing in your pursuit of becoming a sexually confident wife. Working together, you, your husband, and the spiritual leader that serves as a mediator between you and your Higher Power can surely come up with a workable solution to whatever problems may be holding you back.

Even if you hold no religious beliefs at all, a case can still be made that women should feel the freedom to embrace their sexuality and enjoy being sexually confident wives. How so? Because you're a human being, and in case you haven't noticed, it's in every human being's nature to be sexual in some form or fashion. To assume that women shouldn't be sexual is like assuming that a frog shouldn't jump or a bird shouldn't fly.

Focusing on the Common Threads

If two people aren't on the same spiritual plane, it can be a challenge to feel as if you are on the same sexual plane—that's just how intricately connected these two aspects of our being really are. Interfaith marriages can be incredibly challenging, especially if one partner is very devout in their spiritual beliefs and the other holds no particular spiritual belief at all, or one that's considered on the opposite end of the theological spectrum. Much damage can be done by beating a spouse over the head with any religious principles, whether from the Bible, the Torah, the Koran, or others. Such will not enhance sexual intimacy in a marriage but will erect walls that separate. However, respect for each other's spiritual beliefs, regardless of how different they may be from our own, can be a bridge that brings us closer together. If you're involved in an interfaith marriage, I encourage you to focus on the things you do have in common rather than on the things you do not. When we examine humanity closely, especially the sexual aspect, we'll discover that we're far more alike than different. ⊚

Following the Pattern

Everything in the world has a purpose, and a pattern that it naturally and instinctively follows in order to fulfill its purpose. If we examine the pattern that human beings naturally and instinctively follow, you'll notice that we have an undeniable tendency to gravitate over and over again toward four things: eating, drinking, sleeping, and sex. Researchers have identified these as the four "pleasure centers" of the brain—pleasure centers that constantly cry out for satisfaction. This is how humans are wired. Those four pleasure centers are where we live, or at least, where we should be living.

When we grow hungry, we don't feel the need to apologize for eating, right? No one casts a stone at us when we become thirsty. We haven't sinned when we fall asleep at the end of a long day. There's absolutely no shame in experiencing hunger, thirst, or exhaustion. So why should human beings feel shame when our sexual appetites cry out to be fed? Why do we (sometimes subconsciously) fear displeasing the God we worship when we experience a desire for sex? Isn't that how humans are designed by God? Aren't we just following the pattern? Fulfilling our purpose? Yes, we are. And to try to deny that purpose or reinvent that pattern because of the social taboos we've allowed to brainwash our thinking is nothing short of heresy.

So what's a shameless "good girl" to do? Enjoy sexual intimacy within marriage as a sweet foretaste of Heaven, or Nirvana, or whatever you want to call it! Which sounds a lot like what these ladies are doing, even if it took them a while to come around to this way of thinking . . .

- René explains, "I truly love sex, and can make love to my husband without fear, but such wasn't always the case. It used to make me incredibly self-conscious and I'd cower under the sheets, hoping he wouldn't expect anything, or just suffer through the experience so I didn't feel bad about withholding sex from my husband. But then he started reading the Song of Solomon to me in bed. Those passages from the Bible made me feel beautiful—even sexy—as well as worthy of sexual pleasure. It inspired me to begin freely giving myself to my husband, and now I eagerly receive every ounce of pleasure he wants to give me. I'm so honored to know that he does this for me and no other person on earth. And I'm lucky to be the one who gets to give him the same gift in return."

- Blanca writes: "Due to a promiscuous past, I wasn't sure how to control my emotional cravings for attention and affection from men. I thought getting married would change all that, but only a few years after walking down the aisle, I almost walked into an extramarital affair. Your book *Every Woman's Battle* was a lifeline for me during that time. I'm currently in a 12-step recovery group for women struggling to overcome sex and love addictions. As I've connected with these women and realized I am not alone in this battle to remain faithful to my husband, God has taught me that He is ultimately the Lover I've longed for. I always saw God as a distant disciplinarian because that's the kind of relationship I had with my earthly father, but getting to know Him more personally and intimately through the reading of His Word, prayer, and meditation has caused me to fall in love with Him. Learning to lean on God like this and accept His gift of unconditional love and mercy has helped me take the burden of responsibility off my husband's shoulders, and as a result we are much closer than we've ever been in our entire marriage. Our sexual experiences with each other are now a truly beautiful and desired experience for both of us. It's like we're worshipping God together in the most uninhibited way possible—through freely giving ourselves to each other and finding unconditional love, forgiveness, and acceptance in each other's embrace."

- After her thirty-two-year marriage ended, fifty-four-year-old Mary wondered if she'd ever feel comfortable having sex with any other man, especially since her first husband had been her first and only partner. "I began praying that if God had another man for me, that I'd be able to enjoy sex with him without all of the fears and insecurities from my first disastrous marriage hindering me in any way." Mary's second husband is significantly different from her first in that he's not just interested in her sexuality but also in her spirituality. Unlike her previous marriage, they attend worship services together and he often puts his hands on her and prays for her before going to sleep at night. "By the time he says 'amen' I am ready to give my body to him completely!" Mary explains exuberantly.

Indeed, heartfelt prayer for each other is one of the best aphrodisiacs I know of, too, Mary! Each of these women is following the pattern, fulfilling her purpose, connecting both sexually and spiritually to another human being in the deepest, most intimate relationship known to man—the relationship known as marriage.

"A more perfect delight when we be naked in each other's arms clasped together toying with each other's limbs, buried in each other's bodies, struggling, panting, dying for a moment. Shall we not feel then, even then, that there is more in store for us, that those thrilling writhings are but dim shadows of a union which shall be perfect?"

—Susan Chitty, writer

A Foretaste of Heaven

Unless you've taken a vow of celibacy as a nun, your spirituality does not require that you abandon your sexual pleasure. Your sexuality shouldn't require you to abandon your spirituality, either. Consider fully integrating the two.

Don't make the mistake of assuming that integrating your sexuality and spirituality will make for a dull combination. Sacred sex doesn't mean boring sex. Rather, the more spiritually connected two people are, the more intimate, playful, and passionate they can be! Like a chocolate and vanilla swirl ice cream cone, integrating our spirituality and sexuality makes for a delightfully satisfying combination.

Now that I think about it, maybe there's a reason we sometimes shout, "Oh, God! I'm coming!" as we experience orgasm. Perhaps sexual climax brings us closer to God than anything else on earth. Isn't a powerful and pleasurable sexual connection, when freely enjoyed between husband and wife, a sweet foretaste of the connection we'll one day experience in the afterlife? When we can intimately know God as fully as we are known by Him and enjoy basking unashamedly in His presence? For that reason alone, let us overcome any spiritual obstacles holding us back from experiencing our own little slice of Heaven here on earth!

Part 6

A Celebration of
Sexual Confidence

16

Passing the Baton

Daniel's online name was the Prince of Pleasure. Nicole's online name was Sweet Juliet. He began flirting in cyberspace to put some pizzazz in his life. She'd sent him romantic poems revealing her deepest dreams and desires. After six months of interacting over the Internet, they were absolutely smitten with each other.

They finally decided to meet for the first time late one night on a remote beach in France. Sweet Juliet would be wearing white shorts and a pink tank top, and the Prince of Pleasure eagerly anticipated hooking up with the girl of his dreams.

Imagine his shock and horror as he approached her, she turned around, and they suddenly realized they already knew each other! In fact, Sweet Juliet turned out to be Daniel's own *mother*! All Daniel could think was *Oh, my God! It's Mama!*[1]

When I first read the article detailing this unlikely romantic relationship, I was aghast at the irony and felt myself blushing on Nicole's behalf. In fact, I hesitated to tell you this story at all because I realize it's rather mentally disturbing! But something else Daniel was quoted as saying jumped out at me as the real lesson here—the golden nugget that we can all walk away with. After the initial embarrassment wore off, Daniel admitted, "The truth is, I got to see a side of my mom I'd never seen before. I'm grateful for that."[2]

Daniel was *grateful* to have gotten a glimpse of something very precious—a glimpse into his mother's own romantic needs and desires. All of a sudden, Mama wasn't just a mother but rather a human being—a sexual human being with all of the longings and aspirations that come with that role. And ironically, knowing this about his mother actually made her more precious to him.

The Power of Motherhood

Granted, Daniel's view of his mother's sexuality was far too "up close and personal." However, I believe that giving our children (especially our daughters) a clearer glimpse into female sexuality will not only endear us to them all the more, but also pass the baton of sexual confidence to the next generation.

Perhaps you are cringing over the idea that we should be more open about our sexuality with our own children. Why not? Men don't seem to have a problem passing that baton to their sons. What are women afraid of? That we'll set a bad example? I believe the reverse is true. By keeping our own female sexuality such a mystery from the next generation of women, we set them up not to be sexually confident but rather to be sexually self-conscious wives. Just listen to what these adult women have to say about the role their mothers played in their lives.

- Iris writes on a prayer request card at one of my Canadian conferences, "Pray that I can stop blaming my single mother for not being there for me when I needed special guidance during my years of awakening sexuality. I grew up so confused about my sexual desires, and still have a hard time feeling comfortable with them."

- Regina e-mails, "My mother told me just before I married that my husband would expect sex on occasion, and that it was a 'small price to pay' for his happiness, commitment, and provision. As a result, I have a hard time not seeing sex as a dreaded marital duty. I feel like a resentful prostitute who has to just close her eyes and bear it in order to survive."

- Ivy says, "Talking about sex with my mom was nonexistent. It was so taboo that when I got curious, I had to run to friends because the only advice I got from my mom was 'Don't do it or you'll disgrace our family.'"

- Kimberly only recalls her mother telling her, "Sex is like washing dishes. There's just some things in life you have to do even when you don't want to."

- Patricia confided, "When I was growing up, I would have sworn that my parents *never* had sex. There was no inkling of any sexual desire between them. No hand holding. No romantic dates. No locked bedroom doors or Do Not Disturb signs. I always knew they loved each other, but I figured making love was surely another matter. And because I couldn't picture my mother as a sexual woman, I couldn't view myself as a sexual female, either."

> " I blame my mother for my poor sex life. All she told me was 'The man goes on top and the woman underneath.' For three years my husband and I slept on bunk beds."
>
> —Joan Rivers, comedian

Of course, sometimes females run to the opposite end of the spectrum as these women. When our mothers fail to show us that marriage is an enjoyable sexual relationship that's worth the wait, we naturally draw the conclusion that marriage *isn't* where great sex is to be had. *Only single people have good hot sex,* we assume. So as reckless teenagers, college students, or young single women, we often push the envelope, cross the line, and pack all sorts of emotional baggage to drag around the rest of our lives. We may even be tempted to look to an extramarital lover to provide the excitement and whirlwind passion that we don't expect can be found in marriage.

Does going to such lengths in search of sexual fulfillment *make* or *break* a woman's sexual confidence? Speaking from experience, I'd have to say I spent far too many years broken. My own ignorance about female sexuality caused me to lose my innocence at far too young an age, and it took many years and thousands of dollars' worth of counseling to regain the dignity and confidence I lost. However, I refuse to let the same happen to my daughter. I've spent sixteen years painting her a beautiful picture of what sexual confidence looks like in a woman, and I will continue to do so as long as I'm alive.

I hope I can inspire you in this last chapter to do the same, because in this sex-saturated world we live in, it's more important than ever to instill sexual values and a healthy confidence in our children, especially our daughters.

Painting a Vivid Picture

Perhaps you are wondering, *What would sexual confidence look like in a child? They're not even sexually active!* A young female doesn't have to be sexually active to develop all of the characteristics of a sexually confident woman!

I recommend mothers take it step by step, instilling new sexual values at each stage of development. To see what this looks like, let's look at seven ways in which sexual confidence can be fostered throughout each unique season of a child's life.

1. Confidence in Her Sexual Vocabulary

From the earliest stages of development, a child begins communicating about his or her genitals, or the genitals of an opposite sex sibling, or even *your* genitals. I'll never forget showering with my baby daughter during a time when she was just learning animal names. I couldn't help but be shocked and amused when Erin pointed to my crotch and declared, "Squirrel!" I guess she was noticing that I had pubic hair in a place where she didn't. I replied, "No, honey, *vagina!*" I pointed to my vagina, then to hers, and she referred to female genitalia from that day on as a *vagina.* On another day after her baby brother was born, I was changing his diaper when Erin asked, pointing to his penis, "Mommy, why don't I have one of those?" "That's a penis, and girls don't have penises. Girls have vaginas," I replied. Of course, in referring to genitals, moms could say things like "that's a wee-wee," or "Those are your privates," but why? Children will only have to unlearn those terms and learn the proper names later on. Besides, using baby terms instills a sense that there's something inappropriate about talking about our genitals, as if they are dirty or nasty, and they're not. Giving her a proper sexual vocabulary at this early age will give her the confidence to communicate with you when questions arise, which is good, because every little girl will eventually become very curious about sexual matters.

2. Confidence in Her Sexual Curiosity

Do you remember the first time you had questions about sexual issues, like where babies come from? How they get in their mommy's tummy? Or how they come out? Most children wonder about this kind of stuff before they even start kindergarten. I believe if they are mature enough to verbalize the question, they deserve straight answers (which don't include anything about a stork, a watermelon seed, or a "baby fairy"). When children have questions about sexuality, we certainly don't want them to feel as if they have to ask their peers or surf the Internet for answers. We want them to come to us! So how can we make sure that happens? By being proactive! Being the absolute *first* person who ever talks to your child about sex will ensure that you establish yourself as the expert (or "sexpert") in their lives. Begin talking about healthy sexuality before your children start attending school, because there they'll hear all kinds of things from other children. Also, tell your children frequently, "You can ask me anything, and you can use whatever words you need to use in order to ask it!" Why is this important? So they'll have the confidence that they won't get in trouble with you for verbalizing their curiosities. Make sure they know that no topic is off-limits. If they've got questions, you're committed to finding appropriate, straightforward answers. For this reason, it's very helpful to have a medical encyclopedia or a good book about sexual development and character in your home. Thumb through these books together every few months or so. Use portions as bedtime stories and remind your child, "Your curiosity about sex is very natural. As you grow up, you're going to have more and more questions, and I want you to know you can always bring those questions to me. If I don't know the answers, we'll research it together until we find the answers." You'll be exemplifying what it means to be not just a sexually confident wife, but also a sexually confident mom.

"Life in Lubbock, Texas, taught me . . . that sex is the most awful, filthy thing on earth. And you should save it for someone you love."

—*Butch Hancock, singer, songwriter*

---

3. Confidence in Her Beauty and Body Image

Remember one of the main reasons a woman loses her sexual self-confidence? Because of how she feels about her body! And chances are, these feelings don't just come out of nowhere at adulthood. I believe they begin in childhood. I remember watching an *Oprah* show one day about how these teenage girls were absolutely obsessing over their bodies, declaring themselves to be so fat and ugly when in fact there was nothing fat or ugly about them at all. Where did they get such notions? Video cameras in their homes revealed that it was their mothers who often complained about their own bodies in the presence of their daughters, so these young women were merely mimicking what they'd been taught to think and feel. Never bash your shape, size, or outer appearance in the presence of your daughter! You'd never say to a friend, "You've gotten really fat and ugly lately!" So why do we say these things to ourselves, either verbally or silently? Sure, encourage your daughter toward becoming or remaining healthy, but leave "diets" out of the equation. Stock the house with lots of healthy food and snacks so that diets are never necessary. Show her by example what it means to love and respect your body, whether you're a size six or sixteen. When you help her feel good about her body now, you'll set the stage for her to feel good about her body as an adult as well.

4. Confidence in Sexual Boundaries

It's unfortunate that we have to talk to children at such an early age about things such as sexual abuse, but with approximately one-third of women (and many men as well) experiencing sexual abuse in childhood, we can't deny the urgency. To avoid this topic simply sets children up for devastating consequences that could negatively affect their sexual confidence for the rest of their lives. Children are often fondled and kissed and forced to do humiliating things to adults or older children who simply have no regard for anything except their own personal jollies. Your daughters and sons must be aware of their rights to say *no* to anything and everything another person may try to get them to do—not just with strangers, but with any person at all including teachers, friends, babysitters, neighbors, or relatives. Teach them that no one should be allowed to touch them anywhere that a modest bathing suit would cover, and neither should they be asked to touch anyone else where a bathing suit would cover. Also assure them that if someone asks them to do anything like this, they must let you know so that you can protect them in the future.

Not only must our children be taught to avoid becoming the target of inappropriate sexual behavior, but they must also learn to carefully monitor their own sexual desires (yes, girls develop sexual desires too, even *your* daughter!). Reading books together such as *Preparing Your Daughter for Every Woman's Battle* (WaterBrook Press, 2005) and *Preparing Your Son for Every Man's Battle* (WaterBrook Press, 2003) will give you lots of fodder for those kinds of discussions.

Make sure your daughter especially is aware that her sexuality is a blessing, not a curse. In his book *Sex God,* Rob Bell writes:

> Think about the parents of a junior high girl who has just hit puberty and all of a sudden her body has changed in some significant ways, and she's being noticed in ways she wasn't before and now she's starting to notice that she's being noticed. Her parents have to talk to her about all of this. They have to wade into the complexity and confusion and mixed messages that our culture is sending their daughter. If they indulge one way, telling her to use her body to get what she needs and encouraging her to draw as much attention to her body as she can, they're encouraging her to act like an animal. But if they ignore these changes and hope the whole thing just goes away, they're sending her an equally destructive message. They're treating her like an angel. Her sexuality and her body and her beauty are good things. They were given to her by God. Her parents must embrace this and all that comes with it. And they have to teach her how to embrace it in an honorable, dignified way. They must live in the tension and then show her how to do the same.[3]

And living in the tension means overcoming our fear of talking about such intimate issues. Actively engage her in frequent conversations, encouraging her to reserve sexual activity for marriage. By doing so, you'll set her up to become both a sexually confident wife and a sexually healthy individual.

5. Confidence in Her Sexual Health

When your daughter develops breasts and hips, will she know that her body is preparing to make babies someday? When she begins menstruating, will she be well aware of what's happening? Will she know about proper feminine hygiene? How to cope with PMS? When it comes time for her to enjoy sex within marriage, will she know beyond a shadow of a doubt that there's no sexually transmitted disease lurking in her body and waiting to be passed on to her husband? When it's time for her to conceive and give birth to her own children, will she have every chance of a smooth pregnancy without struggling with infertility? Sexual health is a matter that women can't take lightly, including your daughter. I'm shocked at how many female college students I talk to who have never had a gynecological visit, even though many have been sexually active for years! Talk about a dangerous gamble! But even women who aren't sexually active need to have routine exams each year beginning at no later than eighteen years of age (unless a problem arises before then such as erratic periods or pelvic pain). Before she goes off to college, Mom, escort her to your gynecologist for her first pap smear. Help her establish a good relationship with the doctor she'll need to visit every twelve months for the rest of her life. Teach her how to do breast self-exams. Teach her how to be a sexually healthy woman.

6. Confidence in Her Sexual Abilities

One of the biggest concerns that leads teens to experiment with premature, unsafe sexual relationships is that they feel as if they must "practice" in order to be a good lover for their spouse someday. You and I both know that multiple sexual partners doesn't make you a good lover. My husband was a virgin when we married. Basketball legend Magic Johnson had hundreds of sex partners. Which would be my preferred lover? That's a no-brainer. Did Greg know what to do on our honeymoon night? Uh-huh! No complaints from me! The truth is that sex is something that our bodies do naturally. You put a naked man and woman in bed together with no rules or regulations, no guidelines or instructions, and it's amazing how biology takes over and brings them together in such a natural way! But again, let her know she can ask you questions about how sexual relationships work because you want her to have sexual confidence, even as an abstinent single woman. Educate her about how both the male and female body responds sexually, clueing her in about things such as erection, ejaculation, clitoral and G-spot orgasm, and so on. Don't worry that these intimate mother-daughter talks are going to arouse her prematurely. If she's not hearing it from you, no telling what she'll be hearing from someone else on the topic. Remind her that it takes more sexual confidence to walk away from premarital sex than it does to cave in under pressure. Assure her that she doesn't need to practice having sex before marriage to be a great lover. Instead, she needs to practice sexual self-control so that all of her sexual power can be unleashed in her husband's direction come that beautiful honeymoon night!

> "Perhaps the best function of parenthood is to teach the young creature to love with safety, so that it may be able to venture unafraid when later emotion comes; the thwarting of the instinct of love is the root of all sorrow, and not sex only, but divinity itself, is insulted when it is repressed."
> —Freya Stark, travel writer

7. Confidence in Her Baton-Passing Skills

Whenever I ask an audience to raise their hands if their parents educated them about their sexuality, I'm saddened at the response.

Maybe two or three hands out of one hundred go up. How can we feel comfortable talking to our children if we have no model to go by? Granted, it's hard to talk to your children if your parents never talked to you. But there must be one generation that draws the line in the sand and says, "The buck stops here. I'll not allow my child to grow up sexually ignorant and self-conscious. I'm going to raise sexually confident sons and daughters!" And if you're like me, I don't want just my children to be sexually confident spouses. I want that for my grandchildren, too, and for every female and male in my family for generations to come! If that's what we want, there's only one way to get it. Demonstrate what it looks like to pass the baton of sexual confidence from one generation to the next. Then encourage her to do the same with your grandchildren someday.

The Best Gift You Can Give Her

Because sexual and relational values are better *caught* than *taught,* the absolute best gift you can give your daughter is to show her how to love her husband like crazy. How? By loving *your* husband like crazy.

I'll never forget the night that my daughter bestowed upon me one of the best compliments she could have given. Fourteen at the time, Erin asked, "Mom, is it okay that I really, really, really want to have a husband and children someday?" I assured her that this desire is bound up in the heart of most every young woman, and that it was perfectly okay. Then she continued, "And Mom, I want a marriage just like you and Daddy have." My heart did backflips for weeks afterward!

Sadly, of the teens I've polled informally over the past fifteen years, I'd say that more than 90 percent of them say that they *don't* want a marriage like their parents'. Don't let your child fall into that category. Show her what her heart longs for most. Give her hope that with a lot of effort and commitment, a happy, fulfilling marriage is definitely possible. Why? Because most likely, just like my daughter, she aspires to be a wife someday. In an *Oakland Tribune* article entitled "Are Women Giving Up on Marriage?," Jeff Jacoby writes:

> Young Americans look forward to being married: 70 percent of 12th-grade boys and 82 percent of 12th-grade girls describe having a good marriage and family life as "extremely important" to them. Even higher percentages say they expect to marry.
>
> The 60s, the sexual revolution, no-fault divorce, the rise of single motherhood—there is no question that marriage has been through a wringer. Yet our most important social institution remains a social ideal. Boys and girls still aspire to become husbands and wives.[4]

And why shouldn't they? In the book *Case for Marriage: Why Married People Are Happier, Healthier and Better Off Financially,* Linda Waite and Maggie Gallagher clearly illustrate that married people live longer, are happier and wealthier, have more fulfilling sex lives, and raise better-adjusted children than single parents.[5] Do we want our daughters (and sons) to live longer? Be happier? Be wealthier? Have fulfilling sex lives? Raise well-adjusted children? Of course we do! And the best encouragement in that direction is to set a stellar example of what a happily married, sexually confident woman looks like.

So learn to overlook the petty differences that may exist between you and your husband. Commit yourself fully to making this marriage not just survive, but thrive! Accept him. Affirm him. Respect him. Revere him. Romance him. Serve him. Seduce him. Celebrate him. I know he's not perfect, and neither are you, but two imperfect people can still create a very perfect love, and a perfect example of what a deliriously happy marriage looks like.

17

Whipped Cream and a Cherry

always got a kick out of my grandmother and grandfather's playful conversations. They frequently talked of their first date, where he leaned over the restaurant table, touched my grandmother's hand as she perused her menu, and insisted, "Now, Jewel, you order anything you want!" to which she smartly retorted, "I will, thank you, because I can pay for it!"

When we'd play dominoes or cards, Grandpa got rather impatient with the game, especially if Grandmother was taking too long at her turn. After biting his tongue as long as he could, he'd finally erupt, "Come on, now! Either you can or you can't!" She'd snap back, "I *can* play, thank you, and you can *hush* until I do!"

Grandpa looked forward to his nightly dose of ice cream before bed, as did I. Grandmother would get out three crystal dessert dishes and scoop them full of mint chocolate chip ice cream. Grandpa would reach around her to grab his bowl, but she'd always smack his hand and say, "It's not done yet!" Then she'd get out the spray whipped cream, create a swirly dollop, and top it off with a maraschino cherry. Grandpa would roll his eyes and say, "I don't need fancy—I just need my ice cream!" But it just wasn't done until Grandmother added her loving finishing touch.

As I began this last section, I asked myself, "What kind of loving finishing touches do I want to put on this book? What will make it perfectly complete?" Then I remembered in school how I never got as much out of the lectures as I did out of the labs. "Don't *tell* me how to do something, *show* me!" I'd often complain to my professors.

So, as one of my finishing touches, I'd like to *show* you vivid examples of what sexual confidence looks like using testimonies from real women just like you.

"Embracing My Inner Sex Goddess"

After reading the first draft of this manuscript, my twenty-something research assistant, Terrica, e-mailed me, saying, "By just reading the first few chapters, I experienced a seismic shift in my whole attitude about my body, my sexuality, and my marriage. Whereas I've preferred the comfort of a long cotton T-shirt or fuzzy robe after the honeymoon five years ago, I now prefer to walk around the house in as little as possible. My husband says I strut around like a sex goddess, and that he loves it!"

Terrica's right. Underneath every woman's frumpy facade lies an "inner sex goddess" just waiting to be unleashed. Use the fuzzy robes for fetching the paper off the front lawn or packing the children's lunchboxes first thing in the morning, but don't hesitate to slip into something sexier when it's just you and Hubby around.

"Taking Turns"

As Greg and I were leading a marriage conference last year, we were inspired by Lael's testimony about how she and her husband, Kevin, came up with a creative solution to a common sexual struggle. She explained, "Early in our marriage we experienced much tension, as our desire for sexual intimacy differed dramatically. I felt under constant pressure to meet his needs, and he felt hurt and rejected if I wasn't interested in sex all the time. All of that changed when we started taking turns initiating sex. We decided that we would each have up to four days to take our turn initiating. After we made love, it would become the other person's turn. We committed to respond with enthusiasm whenever the other person initiated, and 'hinting around' when it wasn't our turn wasn't allowed.

"We have found over the last few years that when you make a decision to respond positively, the feelings quickly follow. We have so much harmony and joy in our sex life now! My husband loves knowing that all he has to do is give me the 'look' when it is his turn and I'll drop what I'm doing and jump into bed! As for me, I found my sexuality blossomed after the pressure was removed. I love planning ways to make my turn surprising or exciting. I also feel the freedom to initiate a 'quickie' when I don't feel I have a lot to give. Our sex life is now a joyous, exciting part of our marriage that draws us closer together."

Lael has figured out the ultimate goal of sex. It should draw us close to each other and provide a safe refuge for each of us to express our sexual and emotional desires. The only way to reach that goal is to communicate honestly and openly, creatively solving problems that hinder the pleasure and intimacy we each long to experience.

Monique has discovered another form of honest communication that's bolstered her sexual confidence . . .

"Recognizing Eye Candy"

In an e-mail, Monique explains, "A little tactic that has really empowered me to be a sexually confident wife is just being vocal toward my husband rather than waiting for a compliment from him to turn me on. Commenting on how sexy he looks when he's working around the house, telling him it makes me hot to watch him doing physical labor, giving him a once-over and a 'Yum-m-m!' as he walks by, etc. Sometimes just saying these things out loud puts me in the mood. I feel empowered to initiate or pursue him rather than simply being the object of his pursuits, and I'm sure it's a welcome relief on his end. As I'm more proactive and affirming of him, it builds confidence in me!"

Yep, it's true! Sometimes simply giving our husbands what we long to receive ourselves is just as effective an aphrodisiac as being on the receiving end. And if quality time together is something you crave, then giving your husband the gift of a sex retreat is one surefire way to satisfy that craving!

"Scheduling Sex Retreats"

Candace says, "I've always heard how we have to be intentional about making time for the most important things in life, and my marriage is certainly my highest priority. So every few months, we schedule a 'sex retreat.' We go to a nice hotel in the area with the sole purpose of connecting with each other sexually and emotionally. We don't waste a lot of time traveling around, sightseeing, or even going to restaurants or movies, because that's not the goal. We can do that with our kids any day of the week. Our goal on these weekends is to indulge in as much passion and pleasure with each other as possible. We turn off our cell phones and order room service. We play fun games like strip poker or seven minutes in heaven, in which we take turns fulfilling each other's wildest sexual fantasies for seven minutes straight. We sleep in late the next morning and spend the rest of the day trying new techniques and positions. We give each other full-body massages and bask in the Jacuzzi tub together. We might read a good book about improving our sex life or use the digital camera for an intimate photography shoot or to make a fun movie that we can watch together during another round of lovemaking. Anything that turns us on and turns our hearts toward each other, that's the order of the day on our sex retreats!"

Can you imagine how much genuine intimacy you could experience on such a weekend? How much pleasure you could give each other? How bonded you'd feel to each other after such extended quality time together? And what man wouldn't love a getaway weekend like that? Grab your calendar and carve out a weekend soon!

Of course, you don't have to wait until you have a whole weekend together to boggle his sex-loving mind! You can do it anytime, day or night.

"A Dream Come True"

Natalie confesses, "One of my favorite things to do is engage in random middle-of-the-night sex. Men are so sexually sensitive at night, and easily aroused in their sleep. While some people might find it irritating to be woken up, my husband loves it so much that he even lets me set the alarm on the weekends for wee-hour-of-the-morning sex. Or when I go to bed long after him, I often crawl under the sheets and get him fully aroused before he's even fully awake. When he realizes what's going on, then, *it's on!* Talk about passionate! He says it's one of the greatest thrills of his life to wake up and, lo and behold, it isn't a dream! It's a very welcome surprise to him, and a huge confidence booster to me."

You also don't have to wait until nightfall to demonstrate your sexual confidence. Like Tracy, you can do that long before bedtime . . . like while he's still at the office.

"Making an Office Call"

With a look of mischief in her eye, my friend Tracy explained, "Tom recently called from the office saying he really needed to work late on a big project that had to be presented to a VIP client the next day. He assumed I'd be angry about it, but I decided to put my big girl panties on and do something to alleviate his stress. I fed the kids, got a sitter, and drove to his office with a big plate of leftovers. He was so appreciative that I brought him dinner, but that's not the only thing I brought him! I locked his office door, closed the blinds, and stripped down to my black underwear. I invited him to feast on his food at his desk while I climbed underneath and enjoyed a more intimate feast. Within minutes I was out of there so he could keep working on that project. I must have made a good impression, as he frequently calls me during the day and says, 'I keep thinking about that time you . . . I may need to work late again soon, you know?' I know what he's really saying. He's really saying that he loves having a sexually confident wife!"

I'll bet he does. And I'll bet Kelly and Diane's husbands would say the same thing.

"His Own Personal *Playboy*"

Kelly and Diane put their heads together and came up with an idea that goes down in my books as one of the most creative I've ever heard! Kelly writes, "Our husbands turned fifty the same year, so Diane and I wanted to give them each a unique gift they'd never forget. At the local community college that summer, Diane took a photography class and I enrolled in a desktop publishing and graphic design class. After we'd learned lots of cool tricks, we spent several more weeks making birthday presents that would knock our husbands' socks off (and other various articles of clothing as well). We created two magazines—their own personal *Playboys*—full of erotic photos of no one but their own sexy wives. One series had a 'professional' theme, where I was wearing a business suit with unbuttoned silk blouse, push-up bra, short skirt, and no underwear with a bikini wax. Another series was a bikini swimsuit theme by my girlfriend's fenced-in backyard pool. Then there was the sweaty workout series with a body ball, jump rope, and weights, and a 'sexy nightie style show' series of photos. I even included a few articles such as "The Three Most Memorable Sexual Experiences You've Ever Given Me" and "Five Things I'd Love to Do with You When No One Is Watching." Being in the military, sometimes my husband is gone for long periods of time, so he can take this with him and know that he's got a sexually confident wife at home eagerly awaiting his safe return!"

And when a man knows he has a woman like that at home, why would he waste his time looking at or even thinking about any other woman? A well-fed man doesn't feel the need to go looking elsewhere for scraps. He knows where his satisfaction can be found—in *you!*

If At First You Don't Succeed . . .

Maybe you've tried to unleash your inner sex goddess or make his sexual dreams come true only to make a slight fool of yourself—like the woman I heard about years ago who drove to the airport to pick up her husband in nothing but a trench coat, then was asked to remove that coat as she passed through the security gate. I've had a few mishaps of my own, such as the time I walked into our backyard buck naked (and nine months pregnant!), assuming the privacy fence would serve its purpose. I hadn't taken into consideration what would happen if the neighbor kid just happened to be climbing the fence in that moment to see where his soccer ball had landed. But did that keep me from ever walking around my house naked again? Absolutely not. I'm just a little more careful now, that's all.

As I was coming up with a title for this chapter, I was also reminded of the time that Greg and I were on board a cruise ship and we decided that "body sundaes" would be fun to make. Room service delivered all the ice cream, whipped cream, and cherries we'd need for plenty of sugary fun. However, within forty-eight hours I was in the infirmary needing antibiotics for the worst urinary tract infection of my life, which put a screeching halt to all lovemaking activities. Little did I know that sugar wreaks havoc on vaginal chemistry! Did I swear off such intimate oral pleasures? Never! We've just learned to keep sugary treats on less-sensitive areas of the body.

The moral of these embarrassing stories is this: *If at first you don't succeed as a sexually confident wife, try, try, and try again!* When you realize you've taken two steps backwards, pledge to take three steps forward! Let's keep pressing on. Let's overcome every hurdle that holds women back in the bedroom. Let's maximize sexual fulfillment in our marriage, creating the mental, emotional, physical, and spiritual connection we all long to experience in this lifetime.

Acknowledgments

To my husband Greg—without your incredible sensitivity, I'd never have become a sexually confident wife. Thank you for looking beyond my weaknesses to recognize my genuine needs. Your unconditional love is by far my greatest asset in life.

To Erin and Matthew, my awesome children. Thanks for not dying of embarrassment when your friends call me "the Sex Lady." May you enjoy great sex lives with your own spouses someday!

Terrica Smith, thank you for the multitude of hours you invested as my research assistant for this book. I also appreciate how you and Josh tested these theories and confirmed that they indeed bring out the Sex Goddess in a gal.

Finally, special thanks to Michael Palgon and Stacy Creamer at Broadway Books for believing in this book before it was ever written. I appreciate the opportunity to release this message that's been like a fire pent up in my bones.

Notes

1. Where Did Our Confidence Go?

1. Angela Ebron, "The Secret Life of the American Wife," *Family Circle,* October 1, 2005, p. 97.
2. *USA Today* (www.drphil.com)
3. Found at www.nlm.nih.gov/medlineplus/ency/article/001953.htm.
4. Robert W. Birth, Ph.D., Pathways to Pleasure, 2000.
5. Ebron, *Secret Life.*

2. Getting on the Right Track

1. Found at www.everything2.com/index.pl?node_id=94926.
2. Ibid.
3. Found at www.themarriagebed.com/pages/biology/emale/female-oxytocin.shtml.
4. Ibid.
5. Found at www.myhealthsense.com/F020813_womenStress.html.
6. Found at www.everything2.com/index.pl?node_id=94926.

4. Healing the Scars of Sexual Abuse

1. Wendy Maltz, "Sexual Healing from Sexual Abuse: Advice for Adult Survivors," *Selfhelp,* 2007, available at www.selfhelpmagazine.com/articles/sex/healing.html.
2. Carol Tuttle, "Healing from Sexual Abuse," SelfGrowth.com, May 1, 2003, www .selfgrowth.com/articles/Tuttle3.html.

5. Cutting Soul Ties That Bind

1. Robin Norwood, *Daily Meditations for Women Who Love Too Much* (New York: Penguin Putnam, 1997), December 30 meditation.
2. Proverbs 26:11.

7. Befriending the Body Image Bear

1. Kim Gaines Eckert, "Love the Skin You're In," *Today's Christian Woman,* July/ August 2006, p. 14.
2. Found at www.eating-disorder-information.com/bodyimage.asp celebrities.
3. Found at www.avalonhills.org/info/bulimia-key-treatment-elements.html.
4. Eckert, "Love the Skin You're In."
5. Found at gatewaynet.netscape.compuserve.com/news/package.jsp?name=fte/ womenavoidsex/womenavoidsex&floc=GW_home_Thu_04_06.

8. Experiencing the Big "Oh!"

1. Tina S. Miracle, Andrew W. Miracle, and Roy F. Baumeister, *Human Sexuality: Meeting Your Basic Needs* (Upper Saddle River, N.J.: Prentice Hall, 2003), p. 33.
2. Natalie Angier, *Women: An Intimate Geography* (New York: Anchor Books, 1999), p. 63.
3. Robert W. Birth, Ph.D., Pathways to Pleasure, 2000.
4. *Medline Plus Medical Encyclopedia,* September 2002., s.v. "orgasmic dysfunction."

10. Tantalizing Sexual Techniques

1. Malcolm Gladwell, *Blink* (New York: Little, Brown, 2005), p. 206.

11. Maintaining Healthy Boundaries

1. Found at www.bbc.co.uk/relationships/sex_and_sexual_health/enjsex_fantasy .shtml.

2. Sex Bulletin, *Men's Health,* June 2006, p. 50.

3. E. O. Laumann, J. H. Gagnon, R. T. Michael, and S. Michaels, *The Social Organization of Sexuality: Sexual Practices in the United States* (Chicago: University of Chicago Press, 1994).

4. Found at internet-filter-review.toptenreviews.com/internet-pornography-statistics .html.

5. Ibid.

6. Found at www.nymag.com/nightlife/mating/29981.

12. Redefining "Normal"

1. Excerpted from Tina S. Miracle, Andrew W. Miracle, and Roy F. Baumeister, *Human Sexuality: Meeting Your Basic Needs* (Upper Saddle River, N.J.: Prentice Hall, 2003), p. 366.

13. Rising to the Challenge

1. Found at abcnews.go.com/2020/Story?id=123845&page=4.

2. "Four Out of Five People Have an STD," Xpress Online Magazine, San Francisco State University, 2003–2004. Found at xpress.sfsu.edu/archives/ magazine/004317.html.

14. Refueling That Lovin' Feeling

1. Miracle, et al. *Human Sexuality,* p. 465.

15. Overcoming the "Church Lady" Syndrome

1. Found at www.religionnewsblog.com/10963/exploring-links-between-sex-and-spirituality.

2. Philip Yancey, *Designer Sex* (Downer's Grove, Ill.: Intervarsity Press, 2003), p. 24.

16. Passing the Baton

1. Grace Green, "Man Dates Gal on Internet for Six Months—And It Turns Out She's His Mother!" Yahoo! Entertainment, Latest News & Gossip—Weekly World News, December 9, 2005. Found at http://entertainment.tv.yahoo .comnews/wwn/20051209/113414040002p.html

2. Ibid.

3. Rob Bell, *Sex God: Exploring the Endless Connections Between Sexuality and Spirituality* (Grand Rapids, Mich.: Zondervan, 2007), pp. 59–60.

4. Jeff Jacoby, "Are Women Giving Up on Marriage?" *Oakland Tribune,* January 23, 2007.

5. Linda Waite and Maggie Gallagher, *Case for Marriage: Why Married People Are Happier, Healthier and Better Off Financially* (New York: Doubleday, 2001).

We invite you to continue your experience
with *The Sexually Confident Wife*
at our website:

www.sexuallyconfidentwife.com

- Share how you feel about *The Sexually Confident Wife* and read what others are saying.

- Download a Readers' Guide for use in your Book Club.

- Communicate with the author or read Shannon's blog.

- Sign up to receive Shannon's "Hot Tips" e-mail messages.

- Purchase additional copies of *The Sexually Confident Wife*.

- Find out about Shannon's other books on sexuality and spirituality.

For more information about having the author speak to your organization or group, please e-mail us at speaking@sexuallyconfidentwife.com.

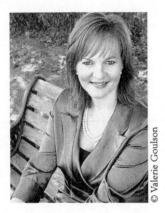

© Valerie Goulson

Shannon Ethridge is an inspirational speaker, counselor, and best-selling author. Her previous books include *Every Woman's Battle* and *Every Young Woman's Battle*. She lives in East Texas with her husband and their two children.